THE CHRONIC STRESS CRISIS

How Stress Is Destroying Your Health
and What You Can Do to Stop It

by

Dr. William G. Timmins

authorHOUSE®

AuthorHouse™
1663 Liberty Drive, Suite 200
Bloomington, IN 47403
www.authorhouse.com
Phone: 1-800-839-8640

© *2009 Dr. William G. Timmins. All rights reserved.*

No part of this book may be reproduced, stored in a retrieval system, or transmitted by any means without the written permission of the author.

First published by AuthorHouse 12/14/2009

ISBN: 978-1-4343-9071-4 (e)
ISBN: 978-1-4343-9070-7 (sc)

Library of Congress Control Number: 2008905877

Printed in the United States of America
Bloomington, Indiana

This book is printed on acid-free paper.

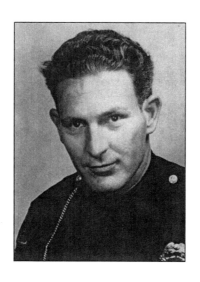

This book is dedicated to the memory of
my father,
Captain William G. Timmins, Sr.

A man with a servant's heart
who taught me unconditional love.

In Memoriam

"Treat the cause, not the symptoms" was a phrase coined by Bill Timmins, my love and husband for more than a decade. Bill would often make the point that mismanaged lifestyle is the root cause of many illnesses, and that any treatment is effective only if accompanied by an accurate diagnosis. As a selfless and devoted physician, Dr. T, as his friends and family fondly referred to him, was constantly seeking to improve and expand upon diagnostic modalities, as the means to determining the root causes of illness. With a solid diagnosis he was confident that he could treat almost any health issue, if the patient committed to a healthy lifestyle.

In his final months of life, Dr. Timmins worked feverishly to complete the book which you hold. *The Chronic Stress Crisis* is his gift to you and your loved ones. It was his wish that everyone, everywhere, could receive its message, so they could experience the joys of a healthy life.

Joan Hunziker, CEO
BioHealth Diagnostics

ONLINE RESOURCES

To locate health professionals utilizing Functional Diagnostic Medicine or to obtain general
recommendations on the ideas, products, and services
discussed in *The Chronic Stress Crisis,* please visit

www.biohealthinfo.com

Contents

Preface by Bryan Timmins	xiii
Foreword by Gerard E. Mullin, MD	xvii
PART I: The Chronic Stress Response	
Chapter 1: My Battle with Chronic Stress	1
Chapter 2: Diagnose and Treat the Cause, Not Just the Symptoms	19
Chapter 3: Your Body and the Chronic Stress Response	43
Chapter 4: Adrenal Syndrome	59
Chapter 5: The Mucosal Barrier: Your First-line Immune Defense	69
PART II: Common Sources of Chronic Stress	
Chapter 6: Bread: The Staff of Life?	79
Chapter 7: Your Body's Uninvited Guests	91
Chapter 8: The Mold Effect	111
Chapter 9: Heavy Metal Toxicity	119
Chapter 10: Chemically Stressed?	133
Chapter 11: Electromagnetic Radiation	149
Chapter 12: Trauma, Inflammation, and Pain	163
PART III: The Four Lifestyle Factors	171
Epilogue: Get the Care You Deserve	205
References	211
Index	225

Preface

In 1992, at the age of 23 and after two months of travel in southern Mexico, I settled back into life in California. Within a few weeks of returning to my routine, I found myself extremely fatigued and depressed, and unable to gain muscle or lose the fat that was developing around my waistline despite efforts to exercise and watch my diet. Frustrated and anxious to regain my vitality, I told my dad, Dr. William Timmins, about my health complaints. He said that "chronic stress" was responsible for my dismal health status and warned that if I did not correct the problems, there could be more severe consequences later on.

This was the first time I had heard the expression "chronic stress." On the surface it seemed self-explanatory—it's a stressful world, filled with responsibilities, hectic schedules, multitasking, and emotional highs and lows. My dad explained further that chronic stress is ANY form of stress to which the body is subject, including externally derived and internally present forms. The stress that I had 24/7, which he suspected resulted from food intolerance and gastrointestinal infections, was impacting my health in a negative way. Add to that any mental stress and/or poor lifestyle habits and the accumulation and complexity of the total load of stress further compromised my body's functioning. All types of stress have the same damaging effect on physiological factors.

Lab testing revealed an assortment of problems. I not only had two parasites living in my gut, I was also intolerant to gluten-containing foods and cow's milk dairy products. Along with that, my adrenal glands were tired. With my hormone system overcompensating to deal with food intolerance and infections, any preexisting problems that I had with my hormones were aggravated.

Dad helped me clean up my diet and treat the infections. He also put me on a regimen of bioidentical hormones to stabilize my adrenal glands. After taking his advice and incorporating lessons about emotional stress and sleep habits, I saw a positive turn in my health. I woke up energized. I was upbeat. I had a sense of calm that had eluded me since childhood! Suddenly, this idea of chronic stress made sense to me: remove and avoid causes of stress! Stress eats away at health. Since I learned that lesson, I have had ups and downs with my health, but one thing that has remained consistent is my immense respect for Dr. William Timmins as a gifted healer and a giving spirit.

This book is the final body of work that he created. In July of 2006, Dr. T passed on after fighting the effects of cancer therapies for three years. In 2003, he was diagnosed with squamous cell carcinoma of the tongue, yet had none of the classic habits or traits of a patient with oral cancer. He did not smoke, drink, or chew tobacco—high risk factors could be ruled out. What caused the tumors to grow? The most direct explanation pointed to a postnasal drip that had been constant for over three decades. An exploratory surgery performed by a biological dentist revealed a tiny crack in his sinus that was severely infected. The crack could be traced to an automobile accident many years prior.

That virtually unnoticeable drip had worn down an area on the base of his tongue, and other lifestyle and environmental factors—which you will read about in the first chapter—precipitated the development of cancer. Dr. T went on to try reputable alternative treatments, primarily autovaccines and low-dose radiation with hyperthermia. The pain and suffering he went through would have killed stronger men. At one point, he wrote on a piece of paper that his entire mouth felt like one giant canker sore! Despite all the agony, he always smiled his famous smile and asked how he could help others.

Ultimately, he beat the cancer. Multiple lab tests confirmed total remission. However, the years of treatments had done irreversible damage to his lungs, and his life could no longer be sustained. It was the last of many health challenges that he endured in his life, and this book was the final act of his educational mission. The concepts behind this book's message could fill volumes, but to best spread the message Dr. Timmins wanted an easy and quick read that would motivate people to act. This book is for you, your family, your friends, and anyone else you care to help move toward a healthy life.

Bryan Timmins
General Manager, BioHealth Diagnostics

Foreword

I was honored when asked to write this foreword on behalf of the author, the deceased Dr. William Timmins. I've had the pleasure of having both a personal and professional relationship with Bill Timmins for 13 years. Like Drs Andrew Weil, Jeffrey Bland, and Jon Kabat-Zin, Bill was a pioneer in what we know today as the field of integrative medicine. I met Bill Timmins in Charleston, West Virginia in 1992, when he was bringing his novel concepts to a population afflicted with environmental illnesses.

He impressed me as a highly educated, experienced, altruistic, and professional individual who was on the cutting edge of transformative healthcare. Bill helped shape my personal growth in self-care and in becoming an integrative medicine professional.

His journey began as a patient afflicted with a severe "incurable" case of environmental illness and ended as a modern-day pioneer of integrative medicine and founder of BioHealth Diagnostics, one of the nation's leading laboratories for functional testing. Over the years, I came to respect Bill's evaluation of the many varied alternative practitioners and types of complementary care during the holistic revolution of the 1990s.

This book, The Chronic Stress Crisis, is a product of Bill's own struggles and accomplishments. It is an enormous contribution to the field of integrative medicine. We live in a society with many inevitable stressors (physical, mental, emotional, environmental), epidemic chronic illness, and the highest per capita spending on healthcare, with poor results. As a nation, the United States is far behind many countries in neonatal mortality and lifespan. The Chronic Stress Crisis outlines the many sources of stress that are a "clear and present danger" to our health. The book not only details the mechanism of how these stressors harm the body, but also outlines how to avoid and overcome these hazards. The many case histories are illustrative and provocative, reflecting Bill's mastery as a clinician.

Those familiar with Functional Diagnostic Medicine will find their understanding deepened by the concepts presented here on integrating mind, body, and spirit to positively influence physiology and improve healthcare outcomes. Those who read this book will discover a one-of-a-kind work on the causes of chronic illness and pearls for overcoming stress and restoring health. Those who come to my office at Johns Hopkins will find a copy of The Chronic Stress Crisis on the bookshelf among books by pioneers and legends such as Walter Willett and others whom I look up to and admire.

Gerard E. Mullin, MD, MHS, CNS, CNSP, FACN, FACP, AGAF, ABHM
Director of Integrative GI Nutrition Services
Division of Gastroenterology and Liver Disease
Johns Hopkins Hospital

PART I

THE CHRONIC STRESS RESPONSE

Chapter 1

My Battle with Chronic Stress

"You will never recover from your illness. Your prognosis is grave at best. We've done all we can for you."

Shocking words, to say the least. A sense of impending doom was setting in. At age 38, I had gone from a robust, energetic 240 pounds to a thin, lethargic 170 pounds on a 6-foot, 5-inch frame in only two months. My body ached. My skin itched. Everything I did and everything I ate seemed to provoke allergic reactions. This doctor and his clinic in Chicago had been my last hope for regaining health. And, now he had declared, "There is no hope."

Deep down, I knew that he was wrong.

Recalling my childhood brings memories of sneezing constantly, struggling with a runny nose, and having itchy eyes, throat, and ears—all classic symptoms of hay fever. Unlike other children who suffered seasonally, I battled these symptoms year 'round. They had been relentless.

Spring and summer brought the greatest attacks, with my suffering so intense that I had to stay inside most of the time. Just opening a window a bit to catch a breeze could provoke extreme allergic reactions. The antihistamines that doctors treated me with worked, sort of. I sneezed less because my sinuses cleared a bit and the itchiness subsided. However, the medicine was so strong that I became drowsy and barely able to function.

I had a tough choice: struggle with the sneezing, watery eyes and itchy skin or take the medications and be free from the symptoms but get dizzy and fatigued. What a terrible catch-22 for a young boy to live with.

Teen Years and Beyond

Throughout my teens, the allergies made life difficult. I struggled to be active athletically and socially. I graduated high school in Alhambra, California in 1961. By this time, my allergies had been reduced to seasonal annoyances. Unsure about a career goal, I decided to work full time and enroll in occasional college courses.

In 1964, I became a California Highway patrolman. To supplement my income, I installed carpeting on my days off. Then a friend invited me to become a business partner in his carpet store franchise. Because the California Highway Patrol offered a one-year leave option with reinstatement, I decided to join the partnership—and never looked back. The carpet store was a success. Eventually, I sold my share in the business and began looking at other opportunities.

In the years that followed, I stepped into a lot of ventures. I started a nightclub, had an import–export company, operated jewelry and real estate businesses, and ran an ad agency. I thrived on having several businesses operating simultaneously. I found time to play rugby and engage in martial arts. Earning four black belts in various martial arts landed me a part-time job with CBS television, where I worked as a bodyguard to celebrities appearing on the programs Challenge of the Sexes and Challenge of the Stars.

During those years, my younger brother, Bob Timmins, was establishing an Adolescent Substance Abuse Program (ASAP) at the Coldwater Canyon Hospital in Los Angeles. Wanting to encourage and support him, I also worked at the hospital part time as a medical technician in the physical medicine unit. During the first two years, I received on-the-job training in occupational therapy, physical therapy, recreational therapy, and biofeedback.

My brother's program met with so much success that it soon expanded to Pasadena Community Hospital. As a result, I was asked to go to Pasadena to head up the new biofeedback unit for ASAP and develop a program for patients in the chronic pain unit. Although it didn't pay well, I immersed myself in this type of work because my businesses and real estate investments were generating income.

While in my thirties and financially comfortable, I decided to commit to the goal of completing my college degree. I liquidated all of my business interests and real estate holdings in Southern California and moved to Oregon with the intent of living in a less stressful environment. I made the move, bought a home, and began college studies full time. Having held some kind of job since age 11, I also wanted to work, and landed a part-time position at a spa as a physical therapist.

After I earned my liberal arts degree, I headed back to Southern California to study Chinese medicine and acupuncture at Pacific College of Oriental Medicine. I didn't stay long, because my interest began shifting toward the study and practice of naturopathy. That's when I took a part-time job working in a medical center and studying naturopathy through an off-site program. Unfortunately, since adequate income became an issue when a number of my investments turned sour, I added a part-time job selling furniture. Sales increased rapidly. Life was good.

Extreme Allergies

A few months after starting the furniture sales job, my skin broke out in hives as I manifested allergic reactions to foods. My other long-standing allergies, dormant for years, erupted as well. When I told doctors about my problem, they tried to convince me it wasn't related to food. I decided to experiment on myself. I started by eliminating different foods from my diet and soon noticed my skin clearing up. Happily, I found a way out of my problem through my own reasoning and experimentation.

My joy was short-lived. Suddenly, for no apparent reason, I began to react to every type of food that I ate and almost everything I smelled and touched. My body eventually reacted to every aspect of my immediate environment: air, food, water, household chemicals, and fragrances. This left me desperate for answers. How was this strange health condition possible?

Within five weeks, I deteriorated from being a strong athlete with 12 percent body fat into a withered shell of my former self. Intense fear set in. Was I going crazy? My anxiety soared when doctors acknowledged that they had no clue what was happening or why. They treated me with steroids and antihistamines, which brought minimal relief and unpleasant side effects, and recommended a dermatology observation unit at Scripps Hospital in La Jolla, California. Emphatically I said, "No." Although I continued losing weight and had hives, ulcerations, and burning and itching all over my body, I refused to subject myself to being a medical guinea pig. I wanted answers, not more shortsighted efforts to make symptoms disappear.

In what became one of many desperate attempts to find out what was happening to my health, I started calling anyone who could offer advice or might know someone who knew something. A fear of impending death came over me. I needed to understand why this was happening.

Keeping Hope Alive

At this time, a priest named Father Doug heard about me from a friend of a friend. He called me and said he believed we had something in common: chemical hypersensitivities. I had never heard the term before and did not understand what Father Doug meant. He suggested that I, like he, had been accidentally exposed to chemicals. The exposure could have been a single time, it could have happened many times, and the chemicals could be breaking down my body's systems. Father Doug recommended a doctor in the area who specialized in treating people suffering from chemical hypersensitivities, more commonly known as environmental illness.

Although I felt grateful for the information, I was perplexed. Having environmental illness meant being exposed to chemicals. If this was true, when and where had the exposure occurred that would have triggered such a devastating effect? Feeling desperate, I made an appointment with the doctor. During a brief consultation, I realized that Father Doug was right.

The symptoms that the doctor described as common to those

with environmental illness matched mine to a T! The question of when and where I had been exposed still baffled me. However, identifying the source of exposure was not that urgent. What mattered was getting treatment. Given the severity of my symptoms and continued weight loss, the doctor determined that an inpatient treatment program would be best. She suggested Henrotin Hospital in Chicago, Illinois. There, I would be under the care of Dr. Theron Randolph. Fortunately, my employer the furniture manufacturer provided good health insurance coverage, allowing me to make the necessary arrangements to get treatment.

I still remember the woeful look on my father's face as he drove me to the airport for my flight to Chicago. He believed that this might be the last time that he would ever see me alive. In contrast, a deep sense of inner calm came over me. Instead of approaching this journey with a fear of disappointment and continued suffering, I had faith that a solution was at hand.

Hospitalized and Losing Hope

When I arrived at Henrotin, I was immediately checked into the "Environmentally Controlled Unit." With my arrival, there were 13 patients in the unit, all suffering from environmental illness.

For the first seven days of my 30-day stay, I was put on a water fast and given enemas daily to help detoxify my body. Then the diagnostic process began. Clinicians gave me small amounts of different foods to determine which ones my body could tolerate without a reaction. Next came testing to identify other allergies and sensitivities. The plan was to treat me with neutralizing dosages of the things to which I tested allergic, a process called provocative desensitization.

The provocative testing began with a small amount of a substance given to me both orally and subcutaneously (under the skin) to see whether it caused a reaction and, if so, the extent of the reaction. Once the team identified my exact sensitivities, they gave me drops under my tongue or injections of tiny amounts of the offending substance. The intent was to neutralize my body's reaction, build a tolerance to the offending substances, and identify at least 12 safe foods for me to eat on a four-day rotation diet. We couldn't find even one safe food! The diet didn't work. The treatments didn't work. Nothing worked.

Even more depressing was my final consultation with Dr. Randolph. He told me, "You will never recover from your environmental illness. Your prognosis is grave at best. We've done all we can for you." He told me I was one of the worst cases he had ever seen. I reacted to everything: foods, chemicals, pollens, molds, and heavy metals. He called me a "classic universal reactor." He also stated that patients with such severe symptoms never recover from environmental illness and have to live the rest of their life in controlled environments.

Despite my disappointment and the uncertainty about my next step, I left Henrotin with an increased understanding of some of the likely causes of my health problems: exposure to heavy metals such as the mercury in my silver/ amalgam fillings and the chemicals in my work environment and home. However, the idea of being forced to live the rest of my life in total isolation was inconceivable. Even if I had the resources to afford such isolation, I was unwilling to live like that.

Dr. William G. Timmins

A "Safe" Environment

I returned to California and went directly to my father's house in Yucaipa, east of Los Angeles. Dad had created a safe room for me that, for the most part, kept me isolated from the external environment. I still had no safe foods to eat and, unfortunately, Yucaipa's air was extremely polluted. I managed rather well until about noon each day, when the smog started rolling in from Los Angeles. I simply couldn't keep the toxic air from seeping into my environment. Although my father was happy to see me, he was baffled and bewildered about my need to live in an isolated and tightly controlled environment. To him, my health seemed to have worsened since I returned from the treatment at Henrotin.

Since I had no safe food, I tried to desensitize myself to foods before eating them. I couldn't introduce a new food into my diet without first trying to neutralize a reaction to that food, a cumbersome two- to three-hour procedure. I used the "teacup" method of desensitization, which involved titrating a food (determining its concentration), then diluting the food to find a neutralizing dose. This would help negate allergic reactions. To do this, I placed a teaspoon of a food substance in a cup of water and stirred it. I then took a teaspoon of water from that cup and placed it in a second cup of water. From that second cup, I again took a teaspoon of the diluted mixture and placed it in yet another cup of water. I continued this process eight to twelve times, which provided a wide range of potencies for just one food. Although this method has helped other people desensitize themselves so they could eat specific foods without reacting to them, the teacup method did not work for me.

Each afternoon as the smog crept in, I drove into the mountains around Big Bear Lake to find cleaner air to breathe. I had actually lined the inside of my car with aluminum foil to reduce outside air from coming in. Eventually my safe haven disappeared as the smog spread, rolling all the way up the ranges to Big Bear Lake. The trees were turning brown from the pollution.

Aside from the air pollution, it was time for me to find another place to live. I realized that the ongoing stress on my father was taking its toll. He tried to help me, yet my misery continued. Dad's despair, anguish, and frustration grew. I knew his health would eventually suffer. In addition, my private disability insurance would soon run out and I couldn't drain my dad's limited resources. Where could I go with no money that would be a safe environment?

Thankfully, Father Doug telephoned to check on my progress and health status. His call was as unexpected and every bit as timely as his first, and my words gushed forth as I told him about my symptoms and suffering. I told him that living in my father's house was no longer an option because of the increased air pollution. I had no safe place to live. Father Doug listened patiently, then invited me to share a house with him in San Clemente, located only a half block from the beach. The air quality would be much better, he promised. Talk about divine intervention! I gratefully accepted his offer.

San Clemente was a huge improvement over anywhere else I had lived; however, I was still disabled and unable to work. Unfortunately, as time went on, I also faced problems with indoor pollution in my new living environment. I felt helpless, hopeless, and emotionally exhausted. I was financially drained, with no safe place of my own to live.

Lacking any notable improvement, I started to believe I would never regain my health or be able to make a living. I briefly contemplated suicide. However, growing up on the streets of East Los Angeles and spending years studying martial arts had made me a fighter—I felt determined not to give up as long as a breath was left in me. I kept fighting every moment, one day at a time. Unfortunately, my current situation was not sustainable. I had to do something, although I had no clear idea what that would be. I just knew that no matter what it took, I would find a way to regain my health.

Perseverance and Faith

In retrospect, I recognize that my faith in God and my self-confidence held me together. My goal was to defeat the thing that gripped me, to fight it with every ounce of my being. Some days it felt like I took one step forward and three steps back. My pain and suffering were horrendous. I battled joint pain, muscle twitching, and seizures. Constipation, cramps, and diarrhea took turns controlling my body. Itchy, burning skin and splitting headaches added to my misery. Intense and often violent muscle spasms blindsided me without warning. My leg muscles would sometimes spasm for hours on end. The pain was so searing, I was convinced that the bones in my legs would break.

I continued to have severe reactions to chemicals and foods. I had to be hooked up to a home oxygen unit most of the time. Despite the oxygen, Heparin, and other treatments to relieve my symptoms—including vitamin C, alkali salts, and various homeopathic remedies—nothing came close to stopping the severe reactions. I began to realize that I needed an even cleaner environment to get a handle on my problems.

While hospitalized at Henrotin, I learned of a woman named Harriet who had been a patient there. After her discharge, Harriet established a community for people with extreme chemical sensitivities. The community was in East San Diego County, along the Mexican border in the little town of Potrero. I met with Harriet and told her about my situation, including that I now had little money and no idea how I would survive.

Harriet understood the suffering of those with environmental illness. She recognized the importance of a clean environment, free from chemicals and pesticides. She knew that only in such a setting could my body begin to detoxify. Despite my inability to pay, Harriet welcomed me into her community.

Harriet fed me organic food, much of which she grew on the property. I slept in an old aluminum trailer that I nearly had to crawl into because of my height. I couldn't even sit up inside the trailer; all I could do was lie down and sleep. In exchange for her kindness, I helped Harriet by doing handyman chores around the property. She displayed great compassion, even with my questionable "fix-it" skills.

Shortly after arriving in Potrero, it became apparent that not even a clean environment would make my symptoms go away. Curiously, now that I lived in one of the cleanest environments I could find, I seemed to suffer even more. How could this be? I thought about this at length. What was wrong?

Then it came to me: I was carrying a toxic environment inside my body; the toxins were embedded in my fat stores and organ systems!

Fortunately, the lack of stress from environmental sources enabled my body to detoxify more. However, the detoxifying process was slow and fraught with symptoms. I experienced body aches, fevers, chills, and painful headaches. The idea of living this way for a long time (possibly the rest of my life) plus being dependent on someone else was not acceptable. I needed to find a more rapid detoxification process. Ultimately, to improve my health, I had to determine the root cause of my illness. I needed to identify and resolve the basic functional weaknesses that kept me in crisis.

Finally, a Clue...

I read everything about environmental illness that I could get my hands on. The books and articles discussed many things relating to exposures—both acute and chronic—to which I had been subject in my work and home environments. Reading them was difficult, not because of the content, but because of the cumbersome process that my health condition necessitated. I had to do all my reading through a strange device called a book box. To use this contraption, I placed my hands inside gloves that were attached to holes drilled in the box. I would then turn on a vacuum to remove any harmful chemical residues that the book might give off, thereby saving me from exposure to the chemicals out-gassing from the books. Regardless of all this research, my illness continued to remain a mystery to my doctors and me.

I contacted people with whom I had worked and grown up, to learn whether they had experienced any environmental illness or chemical hypersensitivity. Luckily, my detective work began to produce results. These people had been exposed to many of the same environmental elements that had made me sick, but none of them suffered from environmental illness. This created more of a puzzle, but it gave me an important clue: Perhaps my internal environment was just as, if not more, significant as my external environment.

Chronic Stress Discovered

I began to study the pioneering work of Hungarian researcher Hans Selye, MD (1907-1982). Dr. Selye developed the theory that "stress is a major cause of disease because *chronic stress* causes long-term chemical changes." Dr. Selye is also quoted as saying, "…stress is not a vague concept, somehow related to the decline in the influence of traditional codes of behavior, dissatisfaction with the world, or the rising cost of living, but rather that it is clearly a definable biological and medical phenomenon whose mechanisms can be objectively identified and with which we can cope much better once we know how to handle it."

Chronic stress is any kind of stress that is repetitive and ongoing. The source can be internal or external. With my research now pointing to the impacts and sources of chronic stress, it appeared that multiple factors could be driving my illness. I identified a lengthy and frightening list of lifestyle, biochemical, and psychological stresses that I had been experiencing for a long time. As I studied the list, I experienced a profound realization: my symptoms paralleled the body's natural responses to chronic stress on the hormone, immune, detoxification, and metabolic systems—as Dr. Selye repeatedly emphasized in relating the profound role of the hormone cortisol, the primary chemical in the body that responds to stress. When cortisol is circulating in unhealthy amounts, all body systems suffer.

Accumulated stress results in what I now recognize as the number one cause of all illness and disease—the *Chronic Stress Response*. The Chronic Stress Response is the body's way of adapting to stress—any kind of stress. Under chronic stress, the response of the brain and hormone system is to produce excess cortisol. Over time, with multiple sources of stress demanding this response, the feedback mechanisms between the brain and the hormone-producing organs begin to erode, depriving all of the body's functional components of vital chemicals and energy. We'll explore the Chronic Stress Response in detail in chapter 3.

With this new understanding I eagerly began a step-by-step process to reduce the chronic stress on my body.

Toxins Inside

Among the dozens of books I read, Hal Huggins's *It's All in Your Head* cornered my attention. Dr. Huggins presents a comprehensive study of the negative effects of mercury amalgam dental fillings. The book convinced me that the metal in my mouth was a serious problem, so I decided that a good starting point on my path to recovery was to have all of my fillings removed. However, my chemical sensitivity made it impossible for me to tolerate any type of anesthetic. Therefore, I drew on what I had been taught during many years of martial arts training: I practiced deep meditation to block the pain during the dental work. My dentist was able to remove 14 mercury amalgam fillings without administering anesthetics.

The next major discovery in my research was the work of Zane Gard, MD, who had developed a sauna detoxification program. It was time to get the toxic chemicals and pesticides out of my body. Living out in the desert had initiated that process, but I couldn't rely upon the desert climate alone. I met with Dr. Gard and he began by testing my blood. One of the blood panels he ran showed a high level of the chlorinated pesticide trans-nonachlor. Decades earlier, the U.S. government had outlawed trans-nonachlor. Manufacturers were prohibited from producing or selling it. However, pesticide companies were allowed to use up the inventory they had. I discovered that this pesticide had been used in the home I had purchased in Oregon, which explained my exposure to it.

Since Dr. Gard had never treated anyone with such high levels of this deadly substance, he approached detoxification slowly and prudently. First, he researched trans-nonachlor and learned that it was known to cause permanent neurological damage. Dr. Gard also had great concern about the many other chemicals that had showed up in my blood tests and consulted with a toxicologist before putting me through his sauna program. When the toxicologist saw my reports, he was at a loss for words. He had no idea why Dr. Gard wanted his input—the toxicologist assumed the test results he had reviewed were for a patient who had died!

Finally, I had scientific diagnostic data about the possible cause of my illness—not just theories based on symptoms. I began a 30-day detoxification regimen. I spent six to eight hours each day in saunas heated to 150 to 160 degrees to sweat out the poisons. This detoxification process was more than intense; it was nearly unbearable. However, enduring this process saved my life. My body needed to purge the chemicals and pesticides that were stored deep in my fatty tissues and vital organs.

As the sauna detoxification program progressed, chemicals and poisons flooded out of my body. I experienced up to four intense seizures a day. The detoxification process elicited the same reactions that I had suffered for years, in greater concentration and frequency. Still, as rough as it was, it was the right thing to do. My symptoms were getting worse every day because my body was ridding itself of the terrible toxins and poisons that were killing me. As painful as the seizures were, I felt this would help me get my life back. No amount of discomfort would stop me.

Dr. William G. Timmins

New Beginnings

The time in the desert, the dental work, and the detoxification program were major steps in the beginning of my healing journey. Over time, I was able to gain more insight into my health problems. Fine-tuning diet, exercise, sleep, and stress management became my highest priority every day. Finally, I attained a level of health that enabled me to return to school and work.

I also enrolled in the International University of Naturopathic Sciences. As a result of classes that I had completed, the administration allowed me to test out of some courses, provided that I write a thesis. I wrote my thesis on environmental illness, chemical hypersensitivity, and how these illnesses develop within the body. I taught basic science courses while doing my studies and completed my Doctor of Naturopathy program in three years. I continued to instruct at the university while working full time at the school's medical clinic.

During these years, I was blessed with wonderful colleagues and mentors at the clinic. The medical doctors were not stuck in conventional approaches; rather, they wanted to know, "What drives this condition? What is the underlying cause? How do we discover what is really wrong?" The doctors welcomed my insights from a naturopathic perspective as well as from my ongoing journey toward optimal health.

By being involved in the clinic's research—and keeping my own struggles in mind—I finally understood the causes of my symptoms. In addition to heavy metal and chemical toxicity, I learned that I was intolerant to the gliadin molecule contained in gluten, a protein found in many common grains. Although there were no obvious symptoms, the condition had made me more vulnerable to the toxic effects of chemicals and heavy metals by reducing my tolerance to external stress. Laboratory testing revealed parasitic, bacterial, and fungal infections. These infections were also sources of chronic stress that had weakened my body's system over the years.

Why had I suddenly gone from "good health" to dismal health in a few short months? What had happened? In many ways, the sudden onset of my severe symptoms wasn't really sudden at all. In retrospect, I wasn't as healthy as I thought. Accumulated chronic stress had a profoundly negative effect on my health—physical, mental, and emotional. It is indeed a vicious cycle.

Time for a Change!

Based on my personal experience and 20 years of clinical practice specializing in chronic illness, I believe the time has come for a paradigm shift in healthcare. I survived my own terrible illness and believe that it's important that I tell my story. To avoid unveiling the "mystery" of what causes chronic illness and degenerative disease would be an abdication of my responsibility as a doctor and a human being. To share this message with as many health professionals as possible and to enable them to help their patients, I established a diagnostic laboratory, BioHealth Diagnostics, in 1998, with professional consulting services and national seminars.

Throughout my health crisis, I remained steadfast in my faith. I prayed and promised God that I would help others. I knew that if I could help even one person escape the trap of chronic illness, then my experience would not have been in vain.

The most important lesson from my experience is this: Identifying the sources of chronic stress is the key to diagnosing the cause of virtually any health problem. Identifying the sources of stress— whether they're associated with poor lifestyle habits, infections, food intolerance, or other factors—is the most effective way to isolate the causes and then make an effort to turn off the Chronic Stress Response.

Answers and solutions exist for illnesses—even life-threatening conditions. The key is the diagnosis. If the diagnosis is accurate, the treatment is more likely to be effective. I was fortunate to identify the chronic stresses that had driven my health into the ground before they put me under it!

As I write this book, I think about my incredible journey back to health and am grateful for my second chance at life. I sincerely hope this book will help you improve your vitality, prevent illness, and lengthen your life. If you're already living with chronic illness, you will learn how functional laboratory testing can determine the underlying causes and what you can do to improve your ability to recover.

Chapter 2

Diagnose and Treat the Cause, Not Just the Symptoms

As my story reveals, a variety of stress factors can lead to a Chronic Stress Response, the primary cause of illness and disease. Chronic stress is any kind of stress that is repetitive and ongoing. The source can be internal or external. Sources of chronic stress can be as varied as grief, radiation, food allergies, lack of (or too much) exercise, substance abuse, parasites, injury, keeping late hours, chemical exposure, and so much more. But what must be understood is this: Regardless of the source of stress, the impact on the body is the same. As Dr. Selye discovered, too much of any stress results in maladaptation at the biochemical level. Hormones become imbalanced and depleted, with a downward spiral of physiological dysfunction following that lead. The systems of the body become compromised. Loss of vitality, illness, and disease are the results. We will focus on the specific dynamics of the Chronic Stress Response in the next chapter.

Using laboratory testing to determine the sources and impacts of chronic stress and direct therapies aimed at resolving the causes is a departure from conventional medicine's symptom-focused care. Conventional medicine is strong on acute care and in providing sophisticated diagnostics for isolating major dysfunctions (such as brain, heart, and lung problems), but when it comes to general wellness and prevention and evaluating the body's interrelated systems, it is weak. It needs to be complemented by another philosophy of healing...

As you may recognize from your own experience, mainstream healthcare in America is primarily based on the suppression of symptoms. Medical doctors—as well as many alternative health professionals—provide this type of care. It is entrenched in the minds of patients who expect quick relief, and is supported by health insurance companies and the pharmaceutical industry, whose profitability is largely derived from the sales of drugs that suppress symptoms. Long-term health improvements, which should be the driving force of any healthcare system, are compromised and often sacrificed to a system that thrives on short-term fixes.

An alternative does exist: Functional Diagnostic Medicine.

This discipline incorporates elements of conventional medicine, but emphasizes prevention. Healthcare professionals utilizing Functional Diagnostic Medicine (FDM) critically analyze the body's core functional systems (explained later in this chapter) for dysfunction. Symptoms are addressed, but only if treatment does not impede an accurate diagnosis and is devoid of harmful side effects.

In contrast to conventional medical professionals trained to identify and stifle the symptoms of a disease—I refer to this approach as Medical Intervention—practitioners of FDM use in-depth patient evaluations and laboratory tests to identify lifestyle factors, as well as hidden physical factors, that drive the Chronic Stress Response. Hidden, unseen physical factors are referred to in medical jargon as subclinical; they occur beneath the surface of clinical observation. Subclinical imbalances compromise health despite the absence of symptoms.

If you are like most people, you approach your health with an "if it's not broken, don't fix it" attitude. You may seek professional help only when experiencing intolerable symptoms, or when you're afraid the symptoms might indicate a serious or life-threatening condition. You may gratefully accept your doctor's diagnosis and recommendations for symptomatic care. Indeed, your symptoms may respond favorably to prescription drugs, over-the-counter medications, or natural remedies.

This care may seem like a good thing—after all, we all want to feel better. However, danger lies in suppressing symptoms while the underlying cause goes undiagnosed. The disappearance of pain, skin rash, fatigue, numbness in extremities, heart palpitations, and other symptoms may be only temporary. The fact that you no longer experience any symptoms after treatment does not guarantee that they won't return. Nor does it mean that the cause of the symptoms has been resolved.

For example, you visit your physician complaining of a stomachache. Your doctor recommends a treatment of antacids to quiet your symptoms. Below the surface—outside the watch of her trained eye—the unaddressed cause of your disease process progresses. Although the doctor treated your symptoms, she failed to properly diagnose their source, so the cause has not been addressed.

As a result, the functioning of critical systems upon which your health depends becomes increasingly compromised.

Symptoms as Warning Signs

Symptoms are the outward expression that vital body systems are struggling with stress. In the absence of symptoms, you're unaware that potentially dangerous changes in your health are occurring. You wait until you feel ill before scheduling an appointment with your insurance-approved doctor or visiting an urgent-care clinic.

Your visit typically begins by completing a health questionnaire and being briefly interviewed by a nurse or medical assistant. "What brings you in today? What are your symptoms?" Someone checks your pulse, blood pressure, and temperature. "Are you using any drugs or medications? How long have you had these symptoms? Have they changed? How would you describe the intensity level of your pain?" As you respond to these questions, you're led down a path of shortsighted intervention.

When the doctor enters, she reads the assistant's notes, glances at your health history, listens to your heart and lungs, and palpates your body. Your physician is seeking to classify your symptoms as a specific illness or disease. Based on an evaluation lasting typically no more than 10 to 15 minutes, your doctor makes a "diagnosis" of your condition. Once a diagnosis—in this case, a label—is applied to your symptoms, the doctor can begin "fixing" your problem. Using standard and customary medical protocols, the physician treats the symptoms and may recommend a follow-up visit to determine whether you have been "cured." You have just experienced Medical Intervention.

In cases such as cold and flu, Medical Intervention can get

the job done. Symptomatic relief is sufficient because the body's defenses are usually strong enough to overcome occasional minor ailments. These short-lasting problems tend to respond well, unless the patient has compromised immunity. But, what if your healthcare professional failed to adequately analyze your condition? Stomach pain could indicate a serious bacterial infection like Helicobacter pylori, stomach cancer, or even food poisoning. Would your treatment differ if the doctor had been able to scientifically diagnose exactly why your stomach hurts? Absolutely!

Real-Life Examples of the Danger...

One of my colleagues, a medical doctor, specialized in preventive medicine and nutrition. He experienced ongoing stomach upset. Eventually, his pain and discomfort became intolerable. Medical colleagues ascribed the symptoms to acute indigestion. Conventional medical tests confirmed that he wasn't producing enough hydrochloric acid. Hydrochloric acid stimulates the pancreas to produce digestive enzymes and bile. Without enough of these substances, we cannot adequately digest carbohydrates, proteins, and fats. He supplemented his diet with digestive enzymes and hydrochloric acid to "fix" the problem. The enzymes and supplements brought relief, but only temporarily. Further testing revealed that he had stomach cancer. My colleague died at the age of 34.

What if, instead, his tests had determined why he wasn't producing enough hydrochloric acid? What if the tests had revealed the cause of his hydrochloric acid insufficiency? He may have had a chance to kill the cancer and get a new lease on life.

Many healthcare professionals treat without an accurate diagnosis. They fail to analyze the unseen stresses that are driving the illness. Why does this happen? What are the reasons for this shortsighted diagnostic approach? There are many, but the major ones are:

- Incomplete assessment of the patient.
- Lack of training in FDM and preventative healthcare.
- Refusal of insurance companies and HMOs to reimburse for what they mistakenly label as "nonessential" services.

An incomplete diagnosis results in inaccurate treatment, which in turn prolongs pain and suffering and needlessly increases the cost of healthcare. In the worst-case scenario, as with my young doctor friend, an inadequate diagnosis causes an irreversible decline in health, leading to death.

In another scenario, a patient sees a doctor, complaining about her low libido, fatigue, and memory lapses. This doctor practices standard Medical Intervention. After reviewing her health history, discussing symptoms, and running blood tests, the doctor concludes that she has chronic fatigue. The doctor recommends treating her symptoms according to the standard medical protocol for that condition— typically antidepressants. This patient then decides to get a second opinion from a doctor who follows the FDM model. Using functional lab tests, this doctor discovers that heavy metal toxicity and parasitic infections are contributing causes of her chronic fatigue.

Of course, the treatment protocols for these two diagnoses are worlds apart. The first doctor prescribes medications for the symptoms associated with chronic fatigue. The second doctor, using FDM, addresses the cause of the chronic fatigue by recommending that the patient detoxify the heavy metals from her body and eradicate the parasites. If you were this patient, which approach would you choose?

When you seek assistance from a health professional, you are looking for an educated opinion on what is going on in your body. You want a diagnosis. The purpose of a diagnosis is to direct treatment. But, can treatment be effective when the diagnosis is incomplete or inaccurate? Certainly not, unless we are talking about a simple head cold or similar ailment. With typically short-term ailments, symptomatic treatment might be all you need to feel well. By alleviating or eliminating symptoms, the body is freed of that stress and therefore better able to self-correct without further intervention. However, even in this case, you should ask yourself: Why did I get sick? Though it may seem common, getting sick is not normal. Your immune system, designed to protect you from illness, could be weakened by chronic stress— stress that you can't see and your doctor neglected to diagnose.

Homeostasis: The Body's Natural State of Health

Where does health end and illness begin?

Homeostasis is a condition of dynamic equilibrium inside the body. The body is in a balanced state of being—in other words, healthy. The tissues receive an adequate and constant level of oxygen and nutrients at a cellular level and all systems function in harmony. The nervous system is even-keeled, and all other physiological processes are finely tuned for vitality and resistance to disease. All is well in homeostasis.

We often hear stories about people who were thought to be in excellent health but became sick "one day" and died soon thereafter. Is it possible that a person's health can deteriorate so rapidly? Life threatening illnesses rarely just happen. They usually develop over time—sometimes even decades—before obvious symptoms arise. During that developmental period, chronic stress on the body contributes to the breakdown, setting the stage for disease. The prevalence of cancer and other diseases is evidence that health professionals are failing to recognize and manage the earliest stages of disease. Functional Diagnostic Medicine is the solution to this problem.

The Five Stages of Disorder

Let's consider what I call the Five Stages of Disorder, beginning with a reminder of where you want to be—in homeostasis (in balance). It is important to understand that even in the first stage of disorder, your vitality and ability to resist the damage caused by chronic stress are compromised; however, the signs of this may not be obvious to you.

Homeostasis: A tendency toward equilibrium between the various interdependent systems of the body.

Stage 1 – Deviation from Homeostasis: This is the first stage of disorder. The natural response of the body to any stress is to attempt to return to homeostasis. If this is not possible, compensation takes place and the body moves forward into the second stage of disorder. Deviation from homeostasis can result from a multitude of stresses, including infections, allergies, and toxic exposures.

Stage 2 – Pathophysiology: The functional changes that accompany a particular syndrome or disease. Although the body still attempts to return to homeostasis, it remains in a state of compensation. Normal biochemical functions are disturbed and tissues and organs begin compensating. This is a potential tipping point for the disease process to kick into full gear.

Stage 3 – Pathomorphology: Detrimental changes in the structure of your body accelerate. Cells are dying and yet symptoms may be subtle or nonexistent. Immune function is compromised and there is degeneration of other functional systems. Even in this stage, the body still strives to revert to the previous phase. If unable to do so, it will degenerate with accelerated compensation and unmistakable symptoms will result.

Stage 4 – Symptomatology: In this stage, the body is challenged by symptoms that result from physiological impairment. The body unsuccessfully attempts to return to the previous phase. Its compensatory mechanisms are struggling and dysfunction persists. Lack of improvement further aggravates dysfunction. This is where conventional medicine generally comes into play—when you are feeling lousy.

Stage 5 – Death: The final stage. The body cannot compensate any longer and it cannot sustain the life force. The cumulative effect of stress has subjected the body to suffer a permanent cessation of all vital functions. Heart attack, respiratory failure... such events are common in the transition from stage 4 to stage 5. Many are preventable tragedies. There is nothing sudden about them; they have been developing—often unnoticed—for years.

Understanding the stages of disorder helps to distinguish Medical Intervention from FDM. Medical Intervention focuses on identifying and treating overt symptoms—that is, stage 4. In contrast, FDM focuses on identifying and correcting the sources of the body's stress in stages 1, 2, and 3. With this approach, stresses causing health problems, or likely to cause them in the future, can be eliminated before manifesting as illness.

Dr. William G. Timmins

The Core Functional Systems

In obtaining a meaningful diagnosis, I rely upon lab testing that provides insight into the body's hormonal, immune, gastrointestinal, and detoxification systems. I evaluate these four systems on all of my patients, whether they are very ill, seeking to prevent illness, or just trying to improve their fitness levels. Why these four? Because the quality of their independent and interdependent function has a profound influence on your health. While you should not ignore the standard preventive medical diagnostics—heart and lung tests and colonoscopies, for example—you must complete the diagnostic picture with functional assessments of the four core functional systems. If one or more is compromised, the negative effects spill over to all other systems, creating a chain of events that perpetuate the Chronic Stress Response.

When I work with a patient, I first determine which of the person's systems are healthy and make every attempt to avoid interfering with them, while supporting those that are performing suboptimally. Using laboratory data, I intervene only as much as is necessary to help the body return to homeostasis.

Hormonal System: *Hormones* has become quite the buzzword, especially where weight loss and beauty are concerned. But, hormones are far more important to your health than these concerns represent. In simple terms, hormones are chemical messengers that travel through your bloodstream and enter tissues, where they turn on switches to the genetic machinery that regulates everything from reproduction to emotions to your sense of well-being. Hormones can be thought of as the chemical force that animates you physically, mentally, and emotionally.

Different glands and organs produce hormones. For example, the pancreas produces the hormone insulin, whereas the ovaries produce estrogens and progesterone. Other glands, such as the pituitary and hypothalamus in the brain, secrete hormones such as FSH (follicle stimulating hormone) and LH (luteinizing hormone) that control how much estrogen and progesterone are produced by the ovaries.

Some hormones are composed of large proteins and others of fatty substances derived from cholesterol. An extremely important class derived from cholesterol is the family of hormones termed steroids. Cholesterol is converted to the mother steroid hormone, pregnenolone, which is further converted in the ovaries, testes, and adrenal glands to the other hormones, as directed by signals from the brain.

The steroid family is broken down into five major categories:
1. Estrogens (estradiol, estriol, estrone)
2. Progesterone
3. Androgens (DHEA, testosterone, androstenedione)
4. Glucocorticoids (cortisol, cortisone)
5. Mineralcorticoids (aldosterone)

The steroid hormones are responsible for regulating thousands of different cellular products needed for general cell maintenance and repair as well as reproduction, immune modulation, and brain function. Functional lab testing can assess the balance and output of these critical hormones. The resultant information can direct an intelligent diagnosis and plan of therapy. In this book, we focus on the stress hormone cortisol, its counter-regulator DHEA, and the mother hormone pregnenolone.

Immune System: The human body is always prone to attack by microorganisms, including bacteria and viruses that cause a multitude of diseases, ranging from thrush and the common cold to pneumonia and poliomyelitis. The body's first line of defense against attack is the skin and mucosal barriers. Behind this is a complex defensive system that protects the body against most infections, even when they do penetrate the primary barriers. This system of defense is known as the immune system.

The immune system neutralizes or destroys microorganisms and the toxins created by them wherever they attack the body via the extensive lymphatic system. The spleen, thymus gland, tonsils, bone marrow, and other organs all play a part in the function of the lymphatic system. The network of lymph vessels (capillaries and lymphatics) drains the clear body fluid known as lymph from the tissues into the bloodstream. Special white blood cells that originate in bone marrow, known as lymphocytes, along with antibodies (proteins that neutralize foreign objects), are primarily responsible for carrying out the work of the immune system.

As mentioned, the body's first line of immune defense is called the mucosal barrier. Mucous membranes are an integral part of the immune system. They form a protective barrier between the interior of the body and the outside environment. The mucosal barrier is permeable and allows nutrients into the body while protecting it from infectious agents, allergens, and other harmful substances. If testing reveals that mucosal immunity is impaired, therapies should be initiated to rebuild it.

In addition to evaluating mucosal immunity, I assess cell-mediated immunity and humoral immunity. Cell-mediated immunity works by the activation of specialized cells called macrophages and natural killer cells, which destroy intracellular pathogens (disease-causing microorganisms). Humoral immunity is the aspect of immunity that involves antibodies. Knowing the status of these immune components provides a comprehensive understanding of one's ability to fight infectious agents, defend against toxic exposures such as chemicals and heavy metals, and kill aberrant cancer cells. In this book, I will concentrate on the critical—and often overlooked—gastrointestinal mucosal barrier.

Gastrointestinal System: As you eat, food travels through your esophagus (the passageway that connects your mouth to your stomach). In the stomach, acids and enzymes break down the food into small particles. These are proteins, fats, and carbohydrates. After leaving your stomach, these particles enter the small intestine. This long tube slowly contracts and expands to push the food along through it, while absorbing nutrients that your body uses for energy, growth, and repair. By the time the food reaches the end of the small intestine, almost all of its nutrients have been absorbed. At this point, what's left of the food is mostly water and indigestible waste.

This material then enters the large intestine. Its main job is to remove water from the waste products as they pass through and then recycle this water back to your body. After traveling through this area, the waste is held at the end of the colon in the rectum. It will then leave your body through the anus as stool when you have a bowel movement.

The gastrointestinal (GI) system, which handles your nutritional requirements, also contains a vast mucosal barrier responsible for—in simple terms—keeping the bad out and the good in. The integrity of the GI system is a major focus of my clinical care. Assessing GI health is essential in all patient cases, regardless of conditions or symptoms. Inflammation caused by bacterial and parasitic infections, food intolerances, and other factors can severely damage GI structures and consequently impair innumerable functional processes. GI inflammation alone can send the body into a 24/7 Chronic Stress Response.

Detoxification System: The health of your detoxification system must be considered in any diagnostic workup. It is comprised of the liver, kidneys, skin, and the circulatory, lymphatic, digestive, and respiratory systems. The body has an amazing capacity to process and dispose of toxins. However, like any waste disposal system, it has limitations; the consequences can be disastrous when its capacity to process toxins is hindered. Impaired detoxification deprives the entire body of clean blood supply and, consequently, every cell suffers. Toxins build up in tissues and slow us down.

I always assess the health of the liver, the primary organ of detoxification, to determine its ability to process waste products naturally generated in the body, as well as those generated by toxic exposures. One of the liver's primary functions is filtering blood. Almost two quarts of blood pass through the liver every minute for detoxification. Filtration of toxins is absolutely critical, as the blood from the intestines contains high levels of toxic substances. When working properly, the liver clears 99 percent of the toxins during the first pass. However, when the liver is damaged—especially in hepatitis sufferers and alcoholics—toxin processing is dramatically reduced, increasing chronic stress on all functional systems.

Many of the toxic substances that enter the body are fat-soluble, which means they dissolve only in fatty or oily solutions and not in water. This makes them difficult for the body to excrete. Toxins may be stored for years in fatty tissues, and are released during times of exercise, stress, or fasting. During the release of these toxins, symptoms such as headaches, poor memory, stomach pain, nausea, fatigue, dizziness, and heart palpitations can occur.

If you are serious about preventing health problems or curing existing disorders, you are cheating yourself out of success if you do not focus on getting help for your hormone, immune, detoxification, and gastrointestinal systems. Healthcare providers competent in FDM can help you navigate the relatively complex road to recovery.

Be an Advocate for Your Own Health— Prevention

When health issues are subclinical, how and when can they be identified? By routinely evaluating the health of the core functional systems with lab testing. No matter what the condition, most health problems begin subclinically, without symptoms. Conditions as diverse as chronic fatigue syndrome, depression, insomnia, cancer, and cardiovascular disease all have their beginnings at the subclinical level. If the subclinical issues remain untreated, symptoms eventually appear. As disorder progresses, critical functions become increasingly compromised, further deteriorating health.

You can prevent illness by getting annual checkups that incorporate functional laboratory testing. If FDM had been available when my health had deteriorated, my doctors would have been able to quickly identify the root causes of my illness. I would have recovered more quickly and with substantially less cost, experimentation, and suffering.

The general public is more knowledgeable now than ever about available healthcare options. Information—perhaps too much—on exercise, diet, sleep, and stress management is at our fingertips via the Internet. Treatment protocols, including specific drugs that the pharmaceutical industry wants us to use and natural supplements, often with grandiose claims, are readily available. In fact, we're becoming so knowledgeable about the many facets of healthcare that doctors complain they can't keep pace with their patients.

However, information alone won't keep you healthy or make you well. You must be an advocate for your own health.

- Become aware of your myriad of daily stresses, especially

insidious ones that can undermine your health. Examples include exposure to environmental toxins, stressful work or family situations, and keeping late hours.
- Pay attention to your body and the signs it is giving. If you feel tired, can't think clearly, have a suppressed sex drive, or experience other symptoms, don't accept them as "normal." Your body is telling you that it is not well.
- Realize that your lifestyle choices have the single greatest influence on your health. Harmful influences include smoking, excessive alcohol and caffeine, inadequate sleep, inactivity, poor diet, and mental stress. Part III describes how diet, sleep, exercise, and stress management habits shape the foundation of health.
- Recognize that your choice of doctors largely determines whether you can successfully resolve your health concerns or are likely to find yourself aboard the merry go-round of symptomatic care. Work with a health professional who takes the time to evaluate your health status, history, and lifestyle factors that might be sources of chronic stress.

In my practice, no matter what a patient's health complaints, I offer three options:

1. Treat symptoms with prescription and nonprescription therapies in the hope of achieving partial or complete relief. Although this approach can be effective in relieving temporary pain or discomfort, it seldom stops a serious illness or disease from progressing.
2. Use functional lab tests to discover and treat the cause of a patient's health concerns.
3. Provide symptomatic care while performing lab testing,

provided that I do not interfere with obtaining an accurate diagnosis.

In decades of clinical practice, none of my patients has ever selected the first option. In fact, most choose the second, despite the discomfort their symptoms may cause. Those who select the third option do so because they are suffering from severe pain or other conditions that require immediate intervention. Are you working with a doctor who practices FDM? If so, that's great. If not, I recommend you find one (see www.biohealthinfo.com for resources). That your physician's approach and experience have a significant impact on your long-term health cannot be overemphasized. While you can take control of your health and do your own research, a caring expert with a proven track record makes all the difference.

Ready, Fire, Aim!

Please remember this point: An accurate diagnosis is critical to ensure accurate treatment and, therefore, a positive health outcome. Without an accurate diagnosis, treating symptoms becomes a sloppy game of "Ready, Fire, Aim!"

All too often, conventional medicine addresses health problems by masking underlying conditions. This approach is illogical and has little chance of success. It isn't entirely fair to blame your doctor for this shortsighted approach. Patients expect doctors to help them feel better. This is understandable—no one wants to suffer. Faced with this expectation, many doctors readily treat symptoms to satisfy their patients' demands to get "better" quickly. This suboptimal treatment approach isn't limited to one particular discipline or specialty.

Many chiropractors, naturopathic doctors, nurse practitioners, acupuncturists, nutritionists, holistic healers, and alternative and integrative healthcare professionals are guilty of the same practice. Regardless of training and experience, a large percentage of health professionals treat only symptoms. They address symptoms using homeopathy, herbs, natural therapies, and treatment modalities common to their specialty, but are still treating symptoms without knowing the underlying cause of their patients' ill health. I've discussed this situation with numerous colleagues—including conventional physicians—and most have agreed that symptom focused care is careless. Not surprisingly, the public agrees even more strongly.

To some, it might appear that I'm attacking healthcare professionals across the board. This is not the case. In more than 20 years of laboratory consulting to virtually every type of health professional, I've been impressed with an abundance of integrity, dedication, and talent. My point is simply this: All healthcare professionals must improve their ability to diagnose the causes of illness.

Some of the most thorough diagnostics occur daily in emergency rooms. Emergency room doctors reason that if you're sick enough to arrive there, you must have serious health issues—often life threatening ones—so they "pull out all the stops." I had an opportunity to interview physicians at Scripps Mercy, a teaching hospital in San Diego. I was extremely impressed with Mercy's team of physicians, but saddened to learn that the majority of their patients returned for treatment of the same condition. Crisis management at Mercy is some of the best in the world, yet I wonder how many patients could avoid hospitalization altogether if our healthcare system promoted the practices of FDM.

The Stakes Are High

The majority of Americans are reluctant to seek healthcare except when impaired by illness. Poor insurance coverage, ignorance, time constraints, denial, finances, and other factors are behind this tendency. Delay in seeking care, combined with conventional medicine's inability to diagnose the underlying causes of illness, factors heavily into the increased incidence of serious illness and soaring medical costs. To reverse this trend, I believe our healthcare system must embrace Functional Diagnostic Medicine.

A basic tenet of FDM is to identify and correct subclinical disorders before they manifest in symptoms and illness. Preventive care utilizing functional laboratory assessments may seem a bit costly; however, in the long run, disease prevention is practical and cost effective. After all, chronic illnesses come with high costs: medical expenses, emotional and physical suffering, lost wages, and lifestyle and family disruption.

Ultimately, you are the guardian of your health. No one else can compensate or take blame for poor lifestyle choices. If you trade responsible diet, sleep, exercise, and stress management for irresponsible habits, you're sabotaging your health. Indoor and outdoor environmental pollutants, pesticides, and other toxins found in food and water add to your stress load. Most prescription drugs and over-the-counter medications have side effects that add more stress. Over time, the Chronic Stress Response compromises your core functional systems, shortening and reducing the quality of your life.

I advocate integrating certain aspects of Medical Intervention with FDM to provide the best of care. The divide between these schools of thought is shrinking, thanks to the awareness and actions of health enthusiasts and enlightened medical professionals, but there is a long road ahead. Scientific research and the public interest must prevail over the financial interests that benefit from our increasingly ill society. Simply treating symptoms alone is destined to fall into the annals of medical history along with magic potions and snake oil.

Joe's Story: A Bitter Lesson

The death of a special friend and patient painfully illustrates the significance of addressing stress before the manifestation of symptoms. I met Joe about 20 years ago. He was a very talented writer, a graduate of Juilliard, and a man with amazing wit and intelligence. Like each of us, he had his particular quirks, one of which was that he "hated" doctors. During our first encounter, I was aware that, despite a thick beard, Joe had very sizeable growths covering much of his face and throat. Joe had been diagnosed with cancer, but was unwilling to submit to conventional chemotherapy and radiation treatments. He had decided that he would attempt to self-heal or die trying.

Shortly after meeting, we developed a friendship. Upon learning about the subclinical approach, he decided to entrust his healthcare to a different kind of doctor, me. During our initial consultation, I learned that Joe, in addition to being exposed to various toxins while serving his country in Vietnam, also had a mouth full of toxic metals. His dental work contained the "usual" mercury fillings, as well as nickel and lead from dental care received while in the military more than a decade earlier.

Many of his fillings were in disrepair and actually disintegrating, releasing metals that freely circulated throughout his body and wreaked havoc on cell function. Knowing that environmental toxins, as well as heavy metal poisoning, could be the subclinical stress causing his cancer, I recommended that he have all the metals removed from his mouth, followed by a carefully monitored detoxification program.

I immediately started Joe on a complex regimen of nutritional products to help his body deal with stress, to assist in detoxifying metabolic pathways, and to generally support and rebuild his systems. Within a month after completing his dental work and beginning the detox program, eight of Joe's tumors had shrunk substantially. During the course of the next 12 months, all of his tumors disappeared and his cancer was declared in remission.

Unlike many people, Joe took total responsibility for his health by practicing intelligent lifestyle management. His eating habits appeared flawless and his workout regimen was inspirational. He didn't smoke, drink, use recreational drugs, or use toxic household products. He actively practiced preventive healthcare. Whenever something wasn't right in his body, he would not rest until he knew its cause. Joe had regained his life and he wasn't about to throw away this second chance. As part of his prevention practices, he followed my advice and checked his health status routinely, using various laboratory tests to determine whether his body was experiencing subclinical stress, and if so, the source of that stress.

This routine worked very well for Joe for some time. Then, during a period when he experienced the height of personal and professional accomplishments, his "luck" began to change. Somewhere in the months before a massive and fatal heart attack, Joe's arteries began accumulating plaque. Given his exemplary lifestyle, including meticulous eating habits, it is difficult to understand, on the surface, why he became a victim of heart disease. Some might conclude that the cause was genetic, although there is no evidence to that effect. Perhaps his extreme disdain for conventional medicine played a role; he failed to do regular medical check-ups.

I believe I know why Joe died. About a week before his death, he called me complaining of a series of symptoms that could be indicative of heart disease. I urged him to see a cardiologist immediately, or to check himself into a hospital for diagnosis. Given his busy schedule and disdain of conventional healthcare, he declined to do so despite voicing concerns to several other friends that same week. Joe also asked me what I thought might be driving the symptoms, assuming that they were heart-related. I noted that plaque caused by various infections could be the culprit.

A rudimentary medical explanation is that infections create inflammation, which in turn results in accelerated plaquing. Certain oral infections, including Helicobacter pylori, are implicated in heart disease. I therefore recommended that, in addition to seeking urgent care, Joe test for this infection. That afternoon, unbeknownst to me, he came by my office to pick up the test kit, although as mentioned, he did not seek immediate help in determining if and to what degree he was suffering from a clogged artery. Later that week, the same day that Joe died, I received his test results. They indicated that he had been suffering from a severe H. pylori infection.

My fervent hope is that by telling Joe's story others will be spared his fate. Joe did not have overt symptoms of either heart disease or H. pylori infection until the week that he died. Arteriosclerosis is a disease, a label assigned to a subclinical biological process that does not magically materialize in a week's time. If Joe had heeded his other friends' and my advice to seek the immediate advice of a physician, he might be alive today. If he had maintained his preventive schedule of subclinical testing, including checking for infections such as H. pylori, he might not have suffered from heart disease, because the infection could have been diagnosed and treated before damaging his arteries.

Joe's case demonstrates a common interface between Medical Intervention and the subclinical perspective of Functional Diagnostic Medicine. While Medical Intervention could have saved his life once the problem had become acute, the subclinical approach could have enabled Joe to avoid the disease process entirely.

Chapter 3

Your Body and the Chronic Stress Response

Virtually all health problems share a common source: the effect of ongoing, chronic stress on the body. It is important that you understand the difference between stress, such as situational stress, and chronic stress.

You may identify stress with feelings of exhaustion, anxiety, or emotional fragility, or with similar responses to undesirable situations and conflicts. You might exclaim, "I'm stressed out!" in response to the world around you. These are examples of *situational stress*. However, stress that has become chronic—consistent and ongoing— has a far greater impact on your health and is not as obvious as situational stress. Chronic stress compromises the critical physiological systems that must be balanced to keep your body in homeostasis. When these systems become impaired, physical changes occur that disturb normal function. Like a collapse of dominoes, when one system begins to falter, it stresses the other systems, leading to illness and disease. This is the Chronic Stress Response.

Fundamental to avoiding and resolving chronic illness is an assessment of the sources of chronic stress. With an accurate diagnosis, a physician can recommend therapies and lifestyle changes to minimize and even eliminate the impact and sources of chronic stress. Chronic stress constantly chips away at the body's foundation of health. Vitality is replaced by fatigue, insomnia, anxiety, and other undesirable changes.

There are two types of stress: clinical (obvious) and subclinical (obscure). Typically, we associate clinical stress with lifestyle, including:
- Insufficient or poor quality sleep, rest, and recovery.
- Negatively internalizing mental and emotional events.
- Poor food choices and poor blood sugar control.
- Too much or too little exercise.

You don't need a doctor to identify these sources of stress. Lifestyle factors and the choices you make shape the foundation of your health. And, the longer that chronic stress undermines your core functional systems, the less you are able to compensate for poor lifestyle behaviors. It is a vicious cycle.

Subclinical stress represents the second source of chronic stress. It is internal and hidden from the senses. Like clinical stress, it can do damage without causing obvious symptoms. Examples of subclinical stress include parasitic infections, food intolerances, viruses, environmental toxins, and bacterial overgrowth.

The following are but a few of the obvious and obscure stresses that can lead to degenerative diseases— cancer, autoimmune syndrome, and cardiovascular disease—if they are allowed to persist and become chronic. Do you have any of these stresses in your life? This is a trick question. You may be experiencing some of them and not even know it!

- Air pollution, noise pollution
- Emotional triggers (e.g., anger, anxiety, depression, fear, guilt, worry)
- Excessive or insufficient exercise
- Extreme temperature changes
- Geophysical stress (magnetic fields)
- Gluten intolerance, lactose intolerance, sucrose intolerance
- Infections
- Inflammation
- Keeping late hours
- Light cycle disruption, sleep deprivation
- Malabsorption, maldigestion
- Mental and emotional trauma
- Overwork
- Pain, whiplash, other physical injuries
- Plant, animal, food, mold, and other allergies
- Poor diet
- Surgical procedures
- Toxic exposures (chemicals, heavy metals, household products, radiation)

Dr. William G. Timmins

Chronic Stress Case Study: Mary

Let's look at the case of Mary, a 33-year-old working woman, wife, and mother of a three-year-old child. Mary came to see me after her fatigue had gotten so severe that she could barely get out of bed. She also experienced indigestion every time she ate. In reviewing Mary's history, I learned that she suffered from "super mom syndrome." She experienced a great deal of stress trying to be a perfect wife, mother, and employee. She even kept a perfectly clean house in her "spare" time.

While she was busy taking care of everyone and everything else, Mary neglected her own health. She ate junk food while on the run, slept poorly, and didn't set aside time to exercise or relax. Basically, she drove herself to exhaustion, collapsing into bed every night. Based on functional lab testing, I learned that she had exhausted adrenal glands and related hormone imbalances, as well as a Helicobacter pylori infection.

Conversations revealed that Mary internalized her mental and emotional stress. She felt that life was out of her control and she was just hanging on for the ride. The Helicobacter pylori infection was creating yet another layer of physiological stress, and a chronic one (24/7) at that! I focused Mary's treatment program on making changes in her lifestyle, along with treating her infection and addressing her hormone dysfunction.

While following the program, Mary committed to taking time to prepare and eat balanced, nutritious meals. She and her husband arranged their schedules to give her time to take a brisk walk for half an hour each day. In addition, Mary made a point to be in bed by 10:00 P.M. to ensure she received adequate rest and recovery. Although making these lifestyle changes was difficult, Mary realized that she needed to let some chores slide and rearrange her priorities. Those decisions, followed by smart lifestyle choices day to day, along with follow-up consultations and testing, helped to renew her strength and resolve and put her back on track for a healthy life. Her story demonstrates that anyone can make informed choices to improve health and lower the risk of chronic illness.

Pregnenolone Steal: The Mechanism of Chronic Stress Response

Had Mary's chronic stress continued, her health would have experienced further degradation. One or more of her core functional systems would have broken down, accelerating the damage done by chronic stress.

Hormone imbalance is the mechanism by which this breakdown occurs. Hormones are chemical substances—often referred to as messengers—produced by glands and organ cells, with specific effects on target cells and organs. An ideal balance of hormones enhances metabolism, energy production, immune function, and other processes critical to health. Hormone imbalance degrades such functions and accelerates the aging process.

Under chronic stress, the adrenal glands increase their output of cortisol—often referred to as the "stress hormone." The principal hormones produced by the adrenal glands—cortisol, dehydroepiandrosterone (DHEA), aldosterone, testosterone, estrogens, and progesterone—share a common precursor, the master hormone called *pregnenolone*. Under stress, your adrenal glands are hyperstimulated and pregnenolone is diverted (stolen) from the pathways that produce the principal hormones. Instead, the pregnenolone is used to produce cortisol.

This diversion of pregnenolone to produce cortisol—called *Pregnenolone Steal*—is an essential safeguard that your body enlists during times of stress. However, because pregnenolone is needed for the production of other hormones, elevated cortisol production reduces its overall output and conversion. Reduced hormone output compromises health. Sleep suffers. You feel exhausted. Libido plunges. Recovery from illness is impaired. Your moods swing, seemingly out of your control. These and other negative outcomes handicap your vitality.

Cortisol is not just the primary hormone that responds to stress. It's also responsible for directing immune function and, in proper balance with DHEA, plays a vital role in carbohydrate metabolism, detoxification, inflammatory response, blood sugar regulation, bone and muscle integrity, and much more. Cortisol also mobilizes stored energy from fat, making it available to the brain and muscles to deal with stressful situations. Evolutionarily speaking, this mechanism evolved to assist humans in dealing with episodic stress, which is both short-term and acute. It wasn't intended to cope with the relentless stress of life in the 21st century.

Saliva tests can measure the levels of free cortisol and DHEA in the body. Free hormones (unbound from proteins in the blood) interact with living tissues and are available to work at the cellular level, making salivary testing the most accurate option for evaluating hormone activity. If testing shows that you have adrenal exhaustion, your health professional can offer treatment plans and lifestyle advice. If left untreated, adrenal dysfunction can lead to a totally debilitating and life-threatening form of adrenal failure known as Addison's disease.

The following is a simplified chart that demonstrates the pathways of steroidal hormone production and Pregnenolone Steal. The small arrows show how pregnenolone is diverted from the pathways that produce the majority of your hormones when it needs to help the body cope with stress by producing cortisol.

Steroidal Hormone Principle Pathways

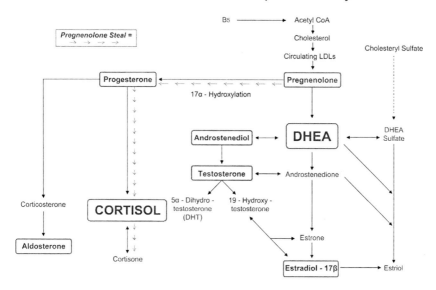

One of the critical hormones that suffers under Pregnenolone Steal is dehydroepiandrosterone (DHEA). As the above chart illustrates, DHEA is the sole precursor and regulator for the production of every steroid and sex hormone in the body. In the Chronic Stress Response, DHEA production declines, as do the downstream hormones. Take testosterone, for example. Men with testosterone deficiency typically experience diminished libido, erectile dysfunction, loss of body hair, depression, and muscle weakness.

Another consequence of Pregnenolone Steal is the diminished output of the hormone progesterone, most commonly associated with women's health and pregnancy. Progesterone is also important for sleep, mood, and other qualities shared by men and women. Progesterone balances the estrogens (estradiol, estriol, and estrone).

It keeps estrogen levels in check by acting as an antagonist to them. Under chronic stress, progesterone levels decline and estrogen dominance results. The result can be menstrual difficulties, increased propensity for miscarriages, unexpected weight gain, anxiety, insomnia, infertility, menopausal conditions, and an increased risk for estrogen-mediated cancers.

In Pregnenolone Steal, the output of the hormone aldosterone is also compromised. Aldosterone is part of the mechanism that your body uses to control blood pressure. Specifically, it controls your body's reabsorption of sodium and water and the excretion of potassium in the kidneys. Proper balance between sodium and potassium is critical to overall electrolyte (mineral) balance, the control of bodily fluids, and the assimilation of nutrients. A deficiency of aldosterone results in your body excreting too much sodium and water in the urine. This causes symptoms such as drowsiness, absentmindedness, salt cravings, and frequent urination.

One of the most important questions to ask when you have any health issue is, "Who or what has stolen my pregnenolone?" In other words, what stresses have become chronic, increasing the demand for cortisol? The sooner you can identify and deal with the offenders, the sooner you can achieve optimal health.

To answer this question, begin by looking at your daily life.

- Could blood sugar control be an issue because of too many simple carbohydrates?
- Could you have an unseen health problem such as subclinical gluten intolerance?
- Do you exercise (too much, too little, not at all)?
- Do you get enough sleep? Are you getting adequate rest to allow your body to truly recover from each day's adventures?

- Do you have silver amalgam fillings in your mouth that are leaking mercury and other toxic metals into your body?
- Do your efforts to maintain your lifestyle create stress?
- Does your work, family life, or relationships cause mental and emotional stress that you can't seem to handle?
- Have you been exposed to chemicals or heavy metals?
- Have you been tested for infections (bacterial, parasitic, fungal, and viral)?
- How well do you eat?

Whatever the stresses that are having an impact on your body, they have one thing in common. When they become chronic, they lead to Pregnenolone Steal, the fundamental mechanism of the Chronic Stress Response.

The Energy Crisis Inside

A major consequence of chronic stress is the impairment of glucose (blood sugar) control, also known as glycemic control. A steady and balanced level of glucose is critical to energy production at the cellular level. If your body is in a Chronic Stress Response, its ability to produce energy is compromised.

If you have an elevated cortisol-to-DHEA ratio, your sensitivity to the pancreatic hormone insulin decreases. Insulin helps control the amount of glucose dissolved in the blood and prevents blood sugar from rising to an unhealthy level. The body's primary energy source becomes severely compromised when sensitivity to insulin is impaired. Your health deteriorates and, aside from common symptoms such as nervousness or fatigue, you might not even be aware of the damage underway.

Another concern related to poor utilization of glucose is called gluconeogenesis. This occurs when your adrenal glands are forced to produce cortisol and your liver is forced to produce cortisone, a hormone with anti-inflammatory and immunity-suppressing properties. The liver's production of cortisone is an adaptive emergency backup system that helps keep your body functioning. Unfortunately, excess production of cortisol and cortisone can destroy muscle tissue. Your brain needs a constant supply of glucose to control your body function via the nervous system. If necessary, your body will destroy heart muscle to get the glucose that your brain requires.

An analogy may be helpful in explaining this. Imagine that your body is a car. As a car, you normally travel at steady speeds. Suddenly, your fuel runs out. Your engine quits and you coast to a stop. Because you're a car, you have no backup system. When the fuel is gone, you simply stop. Your body acts in a similar way, except that it has a backup system. When glucose runs out, your body coasts to a stop, but you have the backup process of gluconeogenesis. It continues to function, but at the price of living off its own "chassis." The topic of glycemic control is focused on in Part III.

Chronic Stress Impairs Immune Defenses

Mucous membranes, known as the mucosal barrier, line your body's cavities and contain immune cells called *secretory immunoglobulins*. Secretory immunoglobulins (sIgA) are released to neutralize undesirable organisms (known as *pathogens*), providing your body's first-line immune defense. The mucosal barrier protects your body's internal environment from pathogens that enter through body cavities, such as the mouth and nose.

If the mucosal barrier is impaired, pathogens can inhabit your body and wreak havoc. Chronic stress adversely affects the mucosal immune system by way of its negative influence on cortisol levels, inflammation control, and antibody production. Under chronic stress, your sIgA production is suppressed because of elevated cortisol. A reduction in sIgA levels heightens the risk for an invasion of opportunistic organisms—namely viruses, parasites, bacteria, fungus, and yeast. Fortunately, lab testing is available to evaluate your mucosal barrier integrity (see www.biohealthinfo.com for lab testing resources). We'll focus on the mucosal barrier in chapter 5.

The Chronic Stress Response also has a negative effect on another type of immune cell called a natural killer (NK) cell. NK cells have two vital jobs: destroying cancer and any infected cells, and protecting against chemicals, poisons, and other infectious agents. If NK cell activity is compromised, sooner or later disastrous consequences will likely occur.

Chronic stress adversely affects other immune cells and chemical messengers. Interleukin 2 (an immune chemical messenger) and T lymphocyte (a class of immune cells) levels both decrease along with a decrease in NK cell levels. Diminished levels of these three key immunological markers are typically seen in people suffering from Acquired Immune Deficiency Syndrome (AIDS), which is caused by the HIV virus. The HIV virus destroys T lymphocytes.

Chronic stress leads to the deterioration of the hormone, immune, detoxification, and gastrointestinal systems. If your body enters this situation, your risk for degenerative diseases increases significantly.

How can you protect yourself?
- Accurately diagnose your sources of chronic stress.
- Address the causes with appropriate treatments and

lifestyle changes.

Taking these steps will increase your odds for living a long and vibrant life. Longevity comes to those who do not sit idly in wait for disease and medical intervention.

Chronic Stress Case Study: Robert

Robert, a 40-year-old single male, suffered from chronic fatigue, fibromyalgia, chronic intestinal yeast infections, and depression. Robert was self-employed and having difficulty working to maintain an income. He had gone for extensive laboratory testing and had seen numerous doctors, all to no avail.

Robert thought that taking human growth hormone might help him. Although his growth hormone profile was at the low end of the reference range for a man his age, I advised him that taking human growth hormone supplements would not address the root cause of his complex health problems. Having struggled with no relief for almost 10 years, Robert felt helpless and had lost hope; he seemed on the verge of a mental, emotional, and physical breakdown.

I did a complete review of his medical history: physical examinations, laboratory tests, current and past symptoms, family history, home environment, hobbies, and so on. While many doctors had run many laboratory tests, there was no logical rationale to the testing. The resulting data were incomplete and, as a result, none of his previous doctors had formed a meaningful diagnosis. Lacking integrated data, the pieces of the puzzle could not be put together, and the source of his problems had remained a mystery for many years. I was looking at a classic example of underdiagnosis and inadequate treatment.

Because none of the laboratory testing ordered by other doctors pointed conclusively to the cause of his chronic fatigue, Robert was simply told that he was "too stressed out." When they were not busy prescribing the latest anxiety drug, some doctors wrote reports that implied he was a hypochondriac.

Seeking answers and desperate to regain his health, Robert went along with one doctor's recommendation to have psychiatric counseling. The psychiatrist emphatically stated that his problems were not psychologically based. Instead, he suggested that Robert's health problems were related to a biochemical issue that was outside the scope of his practice. What Robert really needed was a carefully chosen battery of functional laboratory tests to assess his body's hormone, immune, digestive, and detoxification systems.

It took two weeks to get Robert's test results. As I've seen many times, the results provided the missing links to his health crisis. Robert had advanced adrenal exhaustion and associated low thyroid output, which explained his chronic fatigue. He also had maldigestion, malabsorption, and hypermotility of his small intestine; this meant that food passed through the small intestine so quickly that it couldn't be digested, causing malnutrition and related health issues. The hypermotility was caused by gluten intolerance and two parasitic infections, Giardia lamblia and Cryptosporidium parvum. Robert's Candida yeast overgrowth was also a result of infections and gluten intolerance.

While Candida is normally present in small amounts in a healthy intestine, this opportunistic organism rapidly multiplies to infectious levels in the presence of other infections or conditions that compromise immunity. In addition, Robert's liver detoxification capacity was compromised. Because he had exhausted adrenals, I conducted further testing to measure other hormone levels. As it turned out, Robert's depression was caused by extremely low hormone levels.

At this point, the causes of Robert's symptoms became perfectly clear. Although it took more than six months to resolve all these symptoms, within the first 60 days of treatment, he had improved by 70 to 80 percent. His adrenal function improved dramatically, but he still needed ongoing support because his adrenal glands had been severely depleted. I recommended, as I do with each of my patients, that Robert retest periodically to monitor and validate how he was doing, which would allow him to operate in a preventive mode.

We did a follow-up exam a year later, which was two years from the time that I had first seen Robert. I decided to check his human growth hormone levels again, even though he had not taken human growth hormone. To my surprise, his results came back toward the upper end of the reference range of a healthy 20-year-old!

Restoring healthy function to Robert's hormone, immune, digestive, and detoxification systems allowed him to live a full, healthy life. He is happily married and continues to follow my lifestyle recommendations to optimize his health potential.

"An Ounce of Prevention..."

Most are familiar with Benjamin Franklin's quotation, "An ounce of prevention is worth a pound of cure." Definitely words of wisdom. Unfortunately, most people don't practice prevention. Instead, they seek medical intervention when health problems cause symptoms. Appreciating how the body's critical systems deteriorate under chronic stress strengthens your resolve to practice a healthy lifestyle and engage in preventive healthcare.

It is important to understand that you may feel fine—with no apparent symptoms—even when the Chronic Stress Response is underway. Don't wait until you have developed a complex health problem. The time to prevent and optimize your health is right now.

Chapter 4

Adrenal Syndrome

Adrenal syndrome, also referred to as adrenal exhaustion, is one of the most undiagnosed, misdiagnosed, and mistreated health problems in America today. The degree of its severity ranges from mild dysfunction to total failure of the adrenal glands (known as *Addison's disease*). Because the adrenal glands are responsible for so many critical functions, even a minor impairment in their function can have a negative impact on the entire body. A chronic disruption—one that persists over time—of normal adrenal function can undermine immunity and metabolism, leading to debilitating health conditions.

The adrenals are two walnut-sized glands located just above the kidneys. They are the workhorses of the endocrine (hormone) system. The endocrine system is a group of glands and tissues that release hormones directly into the blood or lymph systems, exerting specific influences on a large number of organs and tissues. Each adrenal gland is divided into two parts: the outer cortex and the inner medulla. The adrenal cortex produces the primary hormones involved in the Chronic Stress Response—cortisol and DHEA.

Why do most physicians fail to recognize this common disorder as the cause—and effect—of many health problems? Besides sheer lack of training and awareness, they often fail in this area because adrenal syndrome can manifest itself in diverse conditions, including neurasthenia (nervous breakdown), hypoglycemia (low blood sugar), anxiety, paranoia, insomnia, depression, trace mineral deficiencies, cerebral allergies, and even food allergies. Some patients are simply told that they're "overly emotional."

This complexity makes in-office diagnosis difficult. In fact, a laboratory test is the only way to scientifically determine how well the adrenal glands are performing. Although this testing is inexpensive and convenient, few doctors are aware of its availability or application. As a result, patients with undiagnosed adrenal exhaustion commonly travel from one doctor to another, seeking to resolve their health problems. The longer the delay in receiving help, the greater the stress on their already taxed adrenals.

What Causes Adrenal Syndrome?

Adrenal syndrome results from chronic stress—conversely, chronic stress promotes adrenal syndrome—and creates an elevated cortisol-to-DHEA ratio from Pregnenolone Steal. Ultimately, exhaustion of the adrenal glands leads to a deficiency of cortisol, DHEA, and other hormones, severely compromising your ability to be healthy and recover from illness.

To understand the cause of adrenal exhaustion, let's consider potential sources of chronic stress. Remember, chronic stress can be either clinical (obvious) or subclinical (obscure). The following list of common clinical consequences and symptoms associated with adrenal exhaustion includes both.

- Alcohol intolerance
- Allergies
- Anxiety
- Bacterial infections
- Blood sugar imbalances
- Craving for sweets
- Depression
- Difficulty building muscle
- Digestive disorders
- Diminished sex drive
- Dizziness upon standing
- Dry and thin skin
- Exhaustion
- Excessive hunger
- Fatigue
- Food allergies
- Fungal infections
- General pain
- Hair loss
- Headaches
- Heart palpitations
- Heavy mental fatigue
- Heavy physical fatigue
- Immune deficiency
- Inability to concentrate
- Indigestion

- Inflammation
- Inhalant allergies
- Irritability
- Joint pain
- Liver disorders
- Low body temperature
- Low blood pressure
- Mood swings
- Pancreatic disorders
- Parasitic infections
- PMS
- Poor memory
- Sinus problems
- Sleep disorders
- Viral infections
- Weakness
- Weight gain in the hips and waist

Absent laboratory testing, misdiagnosis is understandable given the disparate symptoms indicative of adrenal exhaustion. An incorrect assessment usually results in symptoms being treated while the root cause remains undiagnosed.

The common stresses that can cause adrenal syndrome are numerous. When they become chronic in nature, adrenal syndrome can develop. The first sign is persistent fatigue, usually accompanied by associated mood disorders. As the adrenal glands become increasingly exhausted, they fail in their ability to cope with other stresses, further exacerbating the adrenal exhaustion. When experiencing this, many of us feel tired, either all the time or intermittently, no matter what we eat or how well we sleep. Depression is common. Adrenal exhaustion may very well be the culprit of any prolonged or frequent, intermittent fatigue or depression.

Chronic Stress Case Study: Angela

Let's consider the case of Angela, a 32-year-old single career woman who sought my help for fatigue, brain fog, gas and bloating, recurring colds, and PMS symptoms including depression and anxiety. Angela worked in business development for a communications company, had a hectic travel schedule, and found herself dragging by the end of each week. By using functional laboratory tests, I determined that she had an intestinal parasite that was contributing to the Chronic Stress Response. As a result, she suffered from adrenal syndrome. After treating her infection, I used therapeutic doses of botanically derived pregnenolone and B vitamins as part of a program to help balance her hormones.

Within 60 days of beginning her program, Angela's symptoms had dramatically improved. When we retested her adrenal function after 90 days, her cortisol-to-DHEA ratio had dramatically improved and her progesterone levels had normalized. Angela reported that her health problems had not returned.

Sounds simple? It is! I tested her for dysfunction, then delivered the appropriate therapies. Tragically, conventional medicine's standard fix for Angela would have been to prescribe drugs to mask her gastrointestinal symptoms and alter her moods.

The Many Roles of Cortisol and DHEA

I cannot exaggerate the importance of healthy cortisol and DHEA production to your well-being. Too much cortisol can literally burn up the cells of the body; insufficient cortisol production can slow or stall critical processes. What is a healthy cortisol level? Simply put, a healthy level is an adequate amount required to optimally run all the bodily functions under its control. Cortisol and DHEA are produced in the adrenal glands under the stimulation of adrenocorticotropic hormone (ACTH), which is produced by the pituitary gland. The pituitary resides close to the brain, taking all of its cues from the brain's powerhouse, the hypothalamus.

Your nervous system responds to stress by releasing ACTH to stimulate the production of cortisol and DHEA. Interestingly, this occurs regardless of the source of stress. Your body responds to stress in the same way, whether you're being chased by a bear or harboring a parasitic infection in your small intestine. Despite the important function of ACTH, when stress becomes chronic in nature, ACTH is constantly released and, as a result, overstimulates and fatigues the adrenal glands.

Think of it this way. ACTH acts on the adrenals like a jockey whipping a horse to make it run faster. If the jockey ignores the signs that the horse is fatigued and continues to whip the horse, the horse will keep running until it collapses in total exhaustion. Unfortunately, you can expect the same result if you have chronic stress that is out of control.

Let's consider some of the numerous ways that cortisol and DHEA regulate your health.

- **Brain:** High levels of cortisol are lethal to brain neurons and seriously impair memory. Research suggests that excess cortisol production may set up the opportunity for conditions such as dementia and Alzheimer's disease. Cortisol affects the hippocampus, the part of the brain that stores memories. If cortisol is elevated for prolonged periods, the hippocampus does not receive adequate glucose, which it desperately needs to function. Excess cortisol in the brain also slows nerve impulse transmission and can lead to the death of brain cells. In addition, excess cortisol inhibits a brain process critical to memory function called long-term potentiation—a specific communication of neurons.

- **Compensatory mechanism:** One function of cortisol is to break down body tissues, if necessary, to make a steady supply of glucose available to the brain. Cortisol also breaks down body tissues to provide extra glucose to the muscles to help the body cope with stressful situations. However, if cortisol levels are elevated for prolonged periods, the result could be an accelerated catabolic state; the body breaks down its own muscle, connective tissue, and bones.

- **Immunity:** An elevated cortisol-to-DHEA ratio harms the integrity of the body's mucosal barriers. As discussed, mucosal barriers provide the body's first-line immune defense against pathogens seeking to infiltrate the body's internal environment. Cortisol and DHEA direct immune cells called immunocytes that produce the secretory immunoglobulins (as explained in the previous chapter) specific to our mucosal barriers. When the ratio of cortisol to DHEA is elevated, the production of immunocytes—and secretory immunoglobulins—is suppressed, thereby compromising the body's first-line immune defense.

- **Liver:** The adrenal glands play a major role in the liver's ability to detoxify the body from heavy metals, chemicals, poisons, the by-products of infectious agents, and waste products in general. An elevated ratio of cortisol to DHEA impairs the function of detoxification pathways by inhibiting the activity of critical liver enzyme systems.

- **Metabolism:** The adrenal glands oversee the burning and distribution of fat, the metabolism of protein and its subsequent distribution to parts of the body in need of repair and regeneration, and the metabolism of carbohydrates to produce glucose. Many people with excess fat around their hips, thighs, or waist but are normal in weight otherwise. They may even be slender, except for those "problem" areas. Beyond making people uncomfortable about their physique, this kind of accumulation of fat is a telltale sign of adrenal dysfunction, which impairs the body's ability to burn fat.

- **Recovery:** Under healthy conditions, cortisol levels follow a daily circadian rhythm, which means the levels fluctuate on a 24-hour cycle. Cortisol levels peak in the early morning, then gradually decrease over the course of the day, reaching their lowest levels around midnight. The movement of the sun dictates this rhythm. If cortisol levels are too high at night, the body is unable to "shut down" for its physical and psychic regeneration. A high level of cortisol at night inhibits the release of human growth hormone to repair the body's tissues, a process that normally occurs while we sleep.

- **Sex hormones:** The adrenal glands play a major role in producing ovarian hormones. Through the effects of cortisol and DHEA, and in conjunction with hormones released by the pituitary gland, the adrenal glands help "pace" the ovaries. Ovarian pacing means controlling the timing, distribution, and output of the female hormones estrogen and progesterone, which are produced in the ovaries. Without proper cortisol and DHEA levels, female hormones become imbalanced.

- **Thyroid modulation:** The adrenal glands direct the function of the thyroid gland. If you have an abnormally high ratio of cortisol to DHEA, your thyroid output is diminished. In fact, adrenal syndrome is often the underlying cause of hypothyroidism. Many misguided doctors waste their patients' time and money—as well as their health—by focusing solely on the thyroid gland. The patient is often suffering from adrenal fatigue, and treating the adrenal syndrome would resolve the low thyroid. This illustrates the importance of a thorough and accurate diagnosis.

The above examples demonstrate the interdependency of the adrenal glands with other systems and organs of the body. And, this is just the beginning! An infinite amount could be written about the vast influences of cortisol and DHEA on human health. What's important is that you do everything in your power to manage stress—inside and out—and nutritionally support your adrenals to avoid Adrenal Syndrome. Healthy lifestyle choices and Functional Diagnostic Medicine are fundamental to achieving this goal. In the next two chapters we'll explore two of the most critical body systems that are often overlooked in preventive care, as well as when symptoms appear.

Chapter 5

The Mucosal Barrier: Your First-line Immune Defense

The mucosal barrier—your first-line immune defense—refers to all of the mucous membranes that comprise the primary interface between the external environment and the internal environment of the body. Mucosal barriers line the surfaces of your eyes, ears, nose, sinuses, mouth, throat, gastrointestinal tract (from mouth to anus), respiratory tract, urogenital tract, and the vaginal tract.

An analogy can be made between the earth's ozone layer and your body's mucosal barriers. The ozone layer lets the right amount of sunlight through, sustaining life on earth; your mucosal barriers allow nutrients through, sustaining your health. The ozone layer prevents harmful levels of radiation from getting through; the mucosal barriers prevent infectious agents and allergens from invading your body. However, just as the earth has a damaged ozone layer, many of us have compromised mucosal barriers that fail to protect us from infectious agents, allergens, and other harmful substances.

I am frequently asked, "Why does one person get sick while another doesn't when they're both exposed to the same infectious agents?" Typically, people who become ill have compromised first-line immunity. Take the example of anthrax, which caused fears of terrorism shortly after the 9/11 attacks on the United States. Individuals exposed to the anthrax spores without getting ill had healthy mucosal barriers. Those who got ill did not. Their mucosal barriers were unable to encapsulate the spores and eliminate them.

The structures of the mucosal barriers vary in appearance depending on their locations in the body. Perhaps the most important one is the barrier lining your intestines, given its sheer enormity and its role in digestion and immunity.

I won't go into great depth describing the complex components and mechanisms by which the mucosal structures function—although it is a fascinating topic for scientific minds. What is important is that you appreciate their significance and vulnerability when exposed to chronic stress, especially in regards to the gastrointestinal tract.

Secretory IgA to the Rescue

Inflammation, the result of tissue damage caused by influences such as food intolerance and parasitic infection, will erode the structures of your mucosal barrier. A structurally sound mucosal barrier is vital to preventing infection and illness—and not just because it acts as a border through which harmful substances are denied access. It is also a functional component of your immunity.

A healthy mucosal barrier contains adequate amounts of secretory antibodies, which are proteins released to neutralize foreign substances that have entered the body. These mucosal antibodies are known as immunoglobulins, with the most abundant being secretory immunoglobulin A, or secretory IgA.

Secretory IgA represents 73 to 90 percent of the mucosal antibodies produced in the mucous membranes by cells called immunocytes. Less abundant are immunoglobulins M and G. All of these antibodies recognize and neutralize commonly encountered pathogens such as bacteria, fungi, parasites, viruses, and yeast. Secretory IgA also recognizes and processes the proteins in foods. When secretory IgA levels are adequate, food proteins are efficiently processed and the potential for adverse reactions, including allergies, is reduced.

Hormones play an important role in your body's production of secretory IgA. Elevated cortisol and low DHEA create a deficiency of secretory IgA. In addition to suppressing the immunocytes that produce secretory IgA, high cortisol/low DHEA causes a state of "fight-or-flight response." In this state, the body behaves as if under threat, increasing demands for cortisol production and creating a state of Pregnenolone Steal. The longer you remain in fight-or-flight under chronic stress, the longer it takes for the immunocytes to recover and stabilize secretory IgA production.

When stress is high, immune defenses are low.

The Danger of Immune Complexes

Each of the many offending microorganisms in our environment is unique, with its own specific antigens (proteins). The mucosal immune system needs to handle these individual antigens appropriately. When secretory IgA is deficient, the body is unable to properly process microorganisms, resulting in their increased penetration through the gastrointestinal tract and into the bloodstream, where they elicit a systemic immune response.

Your body may become overwhelmed with foreign proteins entering its bloodstream, creating antigen overload. Your systemic immunity creates antibodies that bind to antigens to neutralize them. This combined "complex" of antibody and antigen is called an immune complex or antibody–antigen complex. Accumulation of immune complexes put additional stress on your liver and kidneys, impairing detoxification. Accumulation of immune complexes also accelerate allergy and inflammation, perpetuating a vicious cycle.

Depending on where the immune complexes accumulate, the immune system may no longer be able to differentiate between these complexes and the proteins that make up our own tissues. Large immune complexes make us susceptible to autoimmune conditions—conditions in which the body, in essence, attacks itself—involving whatever tissue they enter. For example, if immune complexes invade the intestinal tract system, there is risk for autoimmune gastrointestinal conditions such as Crohn's disease and inflammatory bowel disease.

The Risky Business of Mucosal Barrier Dysfunction

Because we're often exposed to opportunistic organisms that can cause infections and even disease and death, our first-line immune defense must be healthy. Some of the infectious agents that our mucosal immune defense protects us from are bacteria including Clostridium, Salmonella, and Streptococcus; viruses such as herpes, HIV, influenza, poliomyelitis, rotavirus, and rubella; and intestinal parasites such as Giardia lamblia, Cryptosporidium parvum, Entamoeba histolytica, and Blastocystis hominis.

Parasites have a nasty habit of invading compromised mucosal barriers, eroding their surfaces and causing an inflammatory response, which results in the collapse of the barrier's finger-like projections called villi. Collapsed villi can trap infectious organisms such as parasites in pockets where they thrive, perpetuating a 24/7 Chronic Stress Response and depriving the body of nutrients and immune defenses.

Another common source of mucosal tissue inflammation is reactivity to offensive foods. One of the most prevalent and destructive food molecules is gliadin, found in the glutinous portion of grains like wheat and rye. Intolerance to gliadin is referred to as gluten intolerance and is especially common in those with Northern European ancestry. When the gliadin molecule makes contact with a genetically predisposed individual's mucosal barrier, inflammation results, damaging the barrier. I'll address the topic of gluten intolerance in the next chapter.

If the function of your mucosal barrier is compromised, you are at risk for common gastrointestinal diseases: autoimmune achlorhydria (inability to produce hydrochloric acid), pernicious anemia (a condition in which the body does not make enough red blood cells), villous atrophy (a breakdown of the lining of the intestinal tract leading to intestinal permeability), and infectious clostridium (the primary cause of ulcerative colitis). Moreover, a weak first-line immune defense puts you at risk for a myriad of health problems. It ensures that you remain in a Chronic Stress Response.

Dr. William G. Timmins

Revelations of Research

A study of female monkeys looked at mucosal barrier integrity relative to penetration of HIV into the vaginal mucosal barrier. It showed that HIV could not penetrate a healthy barrier. The mucosal barrier has the ability to defend against the penetration of HIV and virtually any other opportunistic organism.

Another study tested the ability of the mucosal barrier to defend against the aggressive parasite Giardia lamblia. Twelve inmates agreed to drink water loaded with live Giardia organisms. Before they drank the contaminated water, tests were performed to measure their mucosal barrier function.

Nine of the twelve inmates' secretory IgA levels were found to be below normal—evidence of compromised first-line immunity. The other three had normal levels of secretory IgA and were considered to have healthy first-line immunity. The study sought to determine which, if any, of the inmates would be able to defend against the Giardia without having to be treated with antiparasitic drugs.

All twelve inmates became extremely ill; they suffered severe diarrhea, flu-like symptoms, cramps, and fever. Of the nine who had compromised mucosal barriers on initial testing, not one showed an elevated mucosal immune response to the Giardia. They were immediately treated with appropriate medications. The three inmates with strong mucosal immune responses tested negative and were not administered medications, but were closely monitored. Over the next couple of weeks, researchers watched their secretory levels shift from elevated to normal. These men continued to test negative and were without symptoms for the duration of the trial.

These studies illustrate that a healthy mucosal immune system enables a natural immunological response to defend against potentially pathogenic (disease-causing) organisms.

A Strong First-line Immune Defense: It's Up to You

Saliva or blood tests can determine the health of an individual's first-line immune defense. These tests measure secretory IgA levels and reveal antibody levels to specific antigens, providing critical information about the health and function of mucosal barrier immune defense. Although they don't identify specific infections, they do indicate whether or not an active infection is present. Further testing can identify the specific infectious agent, providing a doctor with the information necessary to direct treatment.

In addition to being your primary defense against infections, healthy mucosal immune function can prevent autoimmune disease and support the body's ability to tolerate our toxic world. Under persistent chronic stress, your mucosal immunity breaks down, placing high demands on your systemic immunity, or backup system. This can then overwhelm your systemic immunity, leaving your entire immune system compromised. The sooner you identify and eliminate the causes of chronic stress, the sooner you can prevent and reverse illnesses, be they clinical or subclinical in source.

PART II

Common Sources of Chronic Stress

Chapter 6

Bread: The Staff of Life?

In my clinical practice, gluten intolerance has proven to be the single most prevalent source of chronic stress in my patients. If you are gluten intolerant, one of the most destructive things you can do is consume gluten. You would not willingly inhale car exhaust or drink chlorinated pool water, would you? So why eat foods that contain similarly toxic substances? The answer for many is simple: "I don't feel sick after eating gluten." This hidden or delayed reaction is responsible for a tragic misunderstanding of the risks associated with gluten.

Gluten is the general name used to describe the protein component of wheat, barley, rye, oats, and other cereal grains. It is classified into two groups of proteins: the prolamines and glutelins. The prolamine group, especially its gliadin molecule, appears to be the major culprit in causing celiac disease or celiac sprue—a severe form of gluten intolerance—and subclinical gluten intolerance.

Subclinical gluten intolerance is an immunological/inflammatory response to gluten that can occur without noticeable symptoms, but certainly not without harm. Exposure to gluten in intolerant individuals causes significant chronic stress. Gluten intolerance is not an allergy, despite this common misconception. It is an autoimmune reaction in which the immune system attacks the gliadin polypeptide on the lining of the small intestine, causing tissue damage. The tissue damage triggers inflammation, which stimulates the immune system to respond. This leads to a chronic cycle of inflammation and immune system activation—a classic case of the Chronic Stress Response.

To illustrate how toxic gluten can be, consider the following study. An endoscope was inserted into the small intestine of gluten-intolerant individuals to deliver a tiny gliadin molecule and observe the resulting inflammatory response. The effect? The entire small intestine became inflamed for 10 hours! With this degree of inflammation, mucosal barrier surfaces are damaged and often destroyed. As you learned in Chapter 5, this makes way for malabsorption, intestinal permeability, parasitic infections, and other destructive GI and immune processes. The dominos fall.

The inflammatory reaction to gluten in individuals with celiac sprue is similar to subclinical gluten intolerance, except it is far more severe. The difference is as stark as the difference between sunburn from a day at the beach and third-degree burns on a fire victim. Symptoms of celiac include swollen belly, vomiting, diarrhea, muscle wasting, extreme fatigue, and pale, foul-smelling stools that float because of their high-fat content. People with celiac sprue experience disabling pain when they consume gluten.

The clear symptoms of celiac sprue make this condition relatively easy to diagnose. In addition to its clinical presentation, celiac sprue can be detected by a blood test and confirmed with a biopsy of the small intestine. In contrast, gluten intolerance can be present without any symptoms, or ambivalent symptoms. Gluten intolerance is difficult to diagnose without doing laboratory testing.

Is Gluten Intolerance a Silent Epidemic?

The hereditary aspects of gluten intolerance deserve more recognition by the public and health professionals alike. If you are Caucasian and have ancestors from Northern Europe or Scandinavia, you may have inherited some degree of gluten intolerance. Populations representing other races and cultures have a lower probability of being intolerant, but I have seen people of African, Asian, and other ethnic groups also suffer. In my opinion, based on clinical experience and the limited research available, tens of millions of people suffer from subclinical gluten intolerance, and most are unaware of their condition.

Grains have a rich history. Jared Diamond's book *Guns, Germs and Steel* does a great job of telling the story of how cereal grains—primarily wheat and barley—were exported from their origins in North Africa and made their way through Europe to the United States. But humans are genetically designed to thrive on whatever food grows on their native soil. A lot can be said for eating according to our unique regional and hereditary backgrounds.

More can be said about how financial greed is responsible for "foreign" grains becoming commonplace on United States soil. These grains are more of a commodity than they are nutritious. With emphasis placed on growing and transporting high volumes of grains quickly and cheaply, genetic modifications, additives, nutrient destruction, and pesticides are more common than ever. While good sources of organic and sustainably farmed grains are available, they are more the exception than the norm, and typically one must seek out a specialty store to acquire them.

Case Study: Betty

Betty, a 52-year-old Caucasian woman from New York, became my patient. She had a surprisingly pleasant disposition considering how frustrated she was with her health challenges and the inability of doctors to help. She suffered from chronic fatigue, muscle aches, depression, insomnia, and advanced osteoporosis. She said her health problems began in her early twenties and had worsened over the years, despite many attempts to address them. She had several hospital workups, and no expense was spared to diagnose her health problems.

When doctors were unable to diagnose the cause of her conditions, Betty was labeled a hypochondriac with a psychosomatic disorder, meaning that her physical ailments were of a psychological rather than physical origin. She underwent extensive psychiatric evaluation—to no avail. Prescription drugs failed to help her depression. Gradually, her chronic fatigue, fibromyalgia, depression, insomnia, and osteoporosis worsened. She was yet another victim of Medical Intervention's failure to effectively deal with chronic illness.

Betty became desperate and hopeless. I listened carefully to her tale of woe and reviewed her entire health history. I saw no meaningful clues. At that time, I didn't have the array of functional diagnostic tests that are now in use, but I used what was available to assess Betty's hormone, immune, digestive, and detoxification systems.

The tests revealed a number of issues, which clearly validated that Betty was truly ill. Her health problems weren't all in her mind; she had metabolic imbalances. She suffered from extreme adrenal exhaustion and hypothyroidism, but, unfortunately, because of the unavailability of specific testing, I was unable to diagnose the underlying cause of her hormone imbalances. Like other doctors before me, I started working with her by treating her symptoms—with little success.

I reviewed her chart and noticed that her heritage was mostly Irish. I knew that a high statistical risk existed that she could be celiac, yet she had not shown any of the associated symptoms and there was no family history of celiac sprue. One thing led me to suspect that Betty might have a problem with gluten intolerance: her osteoporosis.

I suggested to Betty that she begin a gluten-free diet. She was happy to try it. The results were totally unexpected. Within 60 days of removing all gluten from her diet, her symptoms disappeared! She no longer had chronic fatigue, depression, fibromyalgia, or problems with sleep, and we later determined that her osteoporosis had stopped advancing. I was amazed and relieved when she told me she was 100 percent asymptomatic. Eliminating gluten definitely improved the quality of her life, and may have saved it.

Betty transitioned easily into menopause by balancing her hormones and using laboratory tests to guide safe hormone supplementation. She's now in her early seventies and enjoys a fully functional life.

Dangerous Grains

The following examples illustrate the high cost of ignoring gluten intolerance and represent just a fraction of the health issues associated with this condition. As I said in the beginning of this chapter, in my clinical practice, gluten intolerance has proven to be the single most prevalent source of chronic stress among my patients.

Dairy and sugar are unwelcome. Lactase and sucrase, two enzymes found in the microvilli (hair-like fibers that cover the villi of the small intestine), digest lactose (the sugar component of dairy products) and sucrose (sugars). When the microvilli are damaged, these enzymes are no longer available in sufficient quantities to properly digest lactose and sucrose. Subsequently, if you are gluten intolerant, you run a high risk of being lactose/ sucrose intolerant as well. This is why your doctor is likely to advise you to eliminate all dairy products from your diet and reduce sugar intake until the microvilli have recovered.

Multiple food allergies escalate. Gluten intolerance, in its tendency to inflame and destroy the gut lining—known as leaky gut syndrome—can allow food antigens to enter the bloodstream. Over time, this overexposure causes the immune system to react, and foods that would otherwise be tolerated can become allergenic. Along with avoiding gluten-containing foods, cow's milk dairy, and soy, a four-day rotation diet will help reverse the damage.

The four-day rotation diet was first introduced by Dr. Herbert Rinkel in 1934. The idea is to structure your food intake to allow your body a period of recovery between subsequent exposures to specific foods that may be causing cyclical food reactions. This practice helps reduce the chance of developing new allergies, encourages diet diversity by providing a wide range of nutritional choices, discourages the overindulgence of one food to compensate for the removal of another, and aids in identifying foods that could be causing problems. When following the rotation diet, a specific food is eaten on a particular day of the rotation and is not eaten again until that day of the rotation comes around again. Four days is generally long enough, but people with chronic constipation may need to cycle longer, until regular bowel movements are achieved.

Good fats and oils are wasted. Inability to properly digest fats and oils results from damage to the microvilli. Microvilli contain lacteals that release a milky substance, which breaks down fats and oils into fine droplets so your body can absorb them. Healthy fats and oils are critical to the function of your entire body, especially the brain, heart, and musculoskeletal system.

Infectious organisms proliferate. When weakened by inflammation, the villi collapse onto one another, creating deep pockets in the mucosal barrier's tissues. Mucus that normally flows through the gastrointestinal tract then fills these pockets and creates mucus plugs. Organisms including bacteria, parasites, and fungi can thrive under the protective cover of these plugs. The mucus plugs also make it difficult, if not impossible, for the immune system or antibiotics to effectively eradicate these organisms.

Nutrients are not absorbed. Gluten intolerance results in severe malabsorption of nutrients, which, if unchecked, leads to all varieties of illnesses associated with malnutrition and especially deficiencies in B12, folate, and iron. Additionally, ongoing irritation and inflammation results in a phenomenon called hypermotility, meaning that food passes through the intestines too quickly. This occurs because everything that enters a damaged small intestine is treated as an irritant, so the body acts to remove the irritation by quickly moving the food through.

Rotting protein contributes to cancer risk. Inadequate digestion of protein, carbohydrates, and fats results from eroded mucosal surfaces. Of particular concern is putrefaction, the enzymatic decomposition of nutrients, especially of proteins, with the production of foul-smelling compounds, such as hydrogen, sulfide, and ammonia compounds. Putrefaction occurs from anaerobic bacteria and fungi acting on incompletely digested proteins that reach the large intestine. The byproducts of putrefaction are known to produce more than 30 carcinogens.

Yeast proliferates and adds to the stress. Because of compromised mucosal barriers, most gluten-intolerant individuals experience a Candida (yeast) problem. Candida, an opportunistic organism, is normally found in the large intestine of a healthy individual in small amounts. When gluten intolerance sets the stage for GI dysfunction, Candida proliferates and invades the mucosal lining of the intestines. My clinical experience has repeatedly validated that this Candida connection may be a contributing factor to conditions such as cancer, osteoporosis, brain disorders, intestinal disease, chronic pain, digestive disorders, and infertility, among others.

Time + Avoidance = Recovery

When it comes to gluten intolerance, time and avoidance of offensive foods are the keys to healing. Fortunately, most people can completely recover by totally eliminating gluten from their diets. A lifetime of avoidance is the only known cure.

Once you stop eating gluten, it can take 60 days or more for the inflammation to subside. The overall damage to the small intestine takes six months or more to heal. Deep pockets of the small intestine eventually return to normal depth and the mucus plugs wash out. Unfortunately, any infectious pathogens trapped in the deep pockets are released and can infect other tissues.

Foods to Avoid on a Gluten-free Diet

Avoidance of offensive foods is the key to healing your gastrointestinal system from the damage caused by gluten. Keep in mind that my recommendations are based on my clinical experience and may conflict with popular opinions regarding some of these foods. Note that cow's milk dairy products are listed. This is because many gluten-intolerant individuals also react to cow's milk proteins because their damaged tissues are unable to produce the enzymes that break down lactose. For those who are not otherwise allergic to dairy, it may be possible, as noted above, to resume the consumption of milk products after the gut has healed. I recommend replacing cow's milk dairy products with goat milk dairy products, which are delicious and healthful alternatives. Other preferred alternatives are foods derived from almonds and hemp.

Proteins similar to gluten can be cross-reactive and must be eliminated from the diet. For example, soy contains a protein that closely resembles the gliadin component of gluten. I recommend that gluten-intolerant individuals avoid all soy products. In fact, as many studies show, there is a strong case to be made for avoiding soy products completely, regardless of your ability to tolerate gluten-containing foods.

Two isoflavones found in soy, genistein and daidzen—the same two promoted by the soy industry for everything from menopause relief to cancer protection—are said to demonstrate toxicity in estrogen-sensitive tissues and in the thyroid gland. High levels of phytic acid in soy reduce assimilation of calcium, magnesium, copper, iron, and zinc. Phytic acid in soy is not neutralized by ordinary preparation methods such as soaking, sprouting, and long, slow cooking. Trypsin inhibitors in soy interfere with protein digestion and may cause pancreatic disorders. In test animals, soy containing trypsin inhibitors stunted growth.

Soy phytoestrogens disrupt endocrine function and have the potential to cause infertility and promote breast cancer in women. They are also potent antithyroid agents that cause hypothyroidism and possibly thyroid cancer. Vitamin B12 analogs in soy are not absorbed and actually increase the body's requirement for B12. Infants exclusively fed soy-based formula have thousands of times more estrogen compounds in their blood than babies fed milk-based formula. Premature development of girls has been linked to the use of soy formula, as has the underdevelopment of males.

While I urge you to do your own research on the reported benefits and risks of consuming soy, I recommend avoiding it. Time and time again, I have seen women and children in particular benefit from removing soy from their diets, with the dominant benefits being improved weight control and emotional stability.

Suggested Foods to Avoid in a Gluten-free Diet
- Arrowroot
- Barley
- Couscous
- Cow's milk dairy
- Kamut
- Oats (Controversial; unless they are explicitly labeled "gluten free," I recommend avoidance.)
- Orzo

- Rye
- Semolina
- Soy
- Spelt
- Triticale
- Wheat

Grains that are considered safe (gluten free) are amaranth, buckwheat, corn, millet, quinoa, rice, sorghum, and teff. That said, I recommend that all grains be avoided for two months or more when following a gluten-free diet. As a side note, some of the healthiest people I have ever known did not eat grains, period. And, moderate or eliminate your consumption of corn and rice. I have seen many patients allergic to these foods.

Beware, as many products on the market are labeled "gluten free" yet contain grains that cross-react with gliadin. I've had patients who failed to get well because they were eating such products. If some of these foods have been staples in your diet, don't fret. You can still enjoy a diet rich in variety with delicious alternatives. An abundance of gluten-free foods and recipes is now available and expanding rapidly (see www.biohealthinfo.com for resources).

Don't Eat another Meal in Ignorance

Are you gluten intolerant? If you don't know, find out! We are now able to diagnose both subclinical gluten intolerance and celiac sprue. Technological breakthroughs have occurred in laboratory testing, allowing either saliva or blood to be analyzed to diagnose these conditions. Barring testing, I encourage you to go on a gluten-free diet for 30 days to see what changes occur in your overall health. Merely removing gluten and cow's milk dairy from the diets of some patients, especially children, has resulted in tremendous improvements in health.

I could share countless tales of how the elimination of gluten and its cross-reactive foods alleviated or resolved a myriad of chronic health conditions. Gluten intolerance significantly undermined my own health. If I had known about gluten earlier in my life, my own saga of chronic illnesses might have been prevented.

Chapter 7

Your Body's Uninvited Guests

Parasites. For many, the word conjures up images of third-world living conditions. The risk of contracting parasites within the United States is mistakenly assumed to be low. After all, just look at all of the government regulations intended to create a safe, hygienic environment. Contrary to appearances, the United States is hardly free of infectious "bugs." In fact, many gastroenterologists specializing in gastric infections declare that this country is experiencing an epidemic of parasitic infections. These microscopic critters are indeed a problem, and when you experience chronic stress, you are particularly vulnerable to invasion and infection, especially in the digestive tract. Parasitic infections increase the demand for cortisol, leading to Pregnenolone Steal and the downward spiral of chronic stress.

A parasite is defined as an organism that grows, feeds, and is sheltered on or in a different organism while contributing nothing to the survival of its host. It stands to reason that organisms foreign to our bodies should be evicted if they take up residence there. However, certain bugs are so common in lab findings that many doctors incorrectly assume that they are a "normal" part of body ecology and therefore ignore measures to remove them. As I have repeatedly stated, in the absence of symptoms, most doctors assume there is no existing or pending health concern. In the case of parasites, this is a dangerous assumption.

In 2004, the chief of the National Institutes of Health's Laboratory for Parasitic Diseases stated that you are more likely to contract a parasitic infection in the United States than in Africa. Consider that this opinion comes from a highly credible medical source. I believe that intestinal parasites are reaching epidemic status, regardless of one's social status or hometown. Factors such as increased international travel, immigration, and imported foods, cause parasites of every variety to thrive here. For example, you no longer have to travel to Mexico to contract Entamoeba histolytica, commonly referred to as Montezuma's Revenge. It is abundant right here in the States.

Some of the most common bugs are:
- *Blastocystis hominis*
- *Clostridium difficile*
- *Cryptosporidium parvum*
- *Dientamoeba fragilis*
- *Entamoeba histolytica*
- *Giardia lamblia*
- *Helicobacter pylori*

Symptoms of exposure to these various bugs range from relatively mild digestive problems, such as diarrhea and heartburn, to severe muscle and tissue damage. In some cases, they can be fatal. One of the most troubling aspects of a parasitic infection is that you may not know you have it. You may experience symptoms only initially or perhaps never; meanwhile parasites continue to rob your body of vital nutrients and destroy cells and even organs. Long-term infections increasingly weaken your first-line immune defense and create a domino effect, further compromising the body's defenses and allowing even more opportunistic organisms to colonize in tissues.

A common consequence of parasitic infections is dysbiosis, the condition in which the hundreds of types of bacteria living in the intestines are out of balance. Although dysbiosis may be caused by factors other than parasites—such as poor diet, antibiotic usage, and stress—the damage done by intestinal infections creates rapid and drastic imbalances. The most well-known imbalance involves the overgrowth of Candida albicans, a normal organism often associated with chronic fatigue and depression. Candida overgrowth should be interpreted as a symptom of an underlying disorder and not the cause of the disorder. Candida yeasts are symbiotic organisms. Yeasts overgrow when conditions are right for them, and they can be a nuisance. You cannot—and would not wish to—get rid of all yeast. You want an ecological balance, with yeast growing at a controlled rate, below the symptom-producing level.

Autoimmunity is another concern. If you host parasites over a long period, your body may not be able to differentiate between them and the healthy tissue in which they reside. This triggers an autoimmune response in which the body attacks itself as if its own tissues are an offending pathogen (an organism that causes disease in another organism). In essence, the antibody process gets confused. Autoimmune responses are often associated with rampant tissue damage, such as in multiple sclerosis and rheumatoid arthritis. However, scientists are discovering that autoimmunity might not be all bad. Some studies suggest that in certain situations, particularly where the nervous system is concerned, autoimmune activity is protective of further damage to the body from specific disease processes. Nonetheless, you want to avoid a condition where your body attacks itself! Avoiding parasites will help you accomplish this goal.

You can contract parasites in numerous ways. Walking barefoot, swimming in public pools, physical intimacy, playing with animals, using restrooms, and even getting an insect bite can expose you. However, eating and drinking contaminated food and water presents the highest risk. Data gathered by the National Resource Defense Council shows that more than 40 million people annually are exposed to Cryptosporidium and Giardia from public water supplies—and this is from water that has been chlorinated and filtered.

Restaurant food is a common source of infection. Parasites are easily spread by staff and patrons. Eating uncooked or undercooked foods and frequenting salad bars and buffets elevates the risk. But, dining out should not be all that concerns you. Inadequately cleaned supermarket fruits and vegetables contain viable parasitic cysts (eggs) or even fully developed organisms. Raw and partially cooked meats can be even worse. Ground meats have especially high contamination rates.

I am not trying to scare you or keep you from enjoying your next meal, but use caution and common sense about what you put into your mouth. This is especially critical if you have a compromised mucosal barrier and cannot adequately defend against infectious agents.

Parasite Case Study: Tom

Tom is a retired medical doctor and PhD. After losing his first wife to cancer, he got involved with integrative medicine and alternative therapies based in nutrition and biochemistry. When I was a young man, Tom was the doctor who treated me for allergies. Thirty years later, I became Tom's doctor.

One day Tom told me he had acquired dysentery while traveling. I sent him a diagnostic test kit to determine whether he had a parasitic infection, because his symptoms suggested that he did. It turned out that he had an acute Entamoeba histolytica (E. histo) infection.

Being a physician, he knew exactly how to treat the infection and called me a couple of weeks later to thank me for helping him identify it. At that time, I said to him, "Tom, keep in mind that even though you had an acute infection and have treated it, E. histo can be tricky and invasive. Be sure to do follow-up testing to confirm that you got rid of it."

A year passed before I heard from him again. One day, I received an urgent call from Tom. He said, "I'm scheduled tomorrow morning for a liver biopsy. I have three abscesses in my liver. I was praying and your name came to me, so I'm calling to ask your advice." I reminded him, "You had an E. histo infection about a year ago. Did you retest to make sure you got rid of it?"

Because all of his symptoms had gone away and he felt fine, he hadn't retested. I explained that if he hadn't eradicated the E. histo infection, his liver abscesses could be amebic abscesses. If they were, a biopsy could result in his death within two to three hours from the release of toxins that would overwhelm his body. Tom cancelled the biopsy and I sent him a diagnostic test kit. As I suspected, his test result for E. histo was positive. Although his initial treatment had controlled his symptoms, it hadn't eliminated the infection, which had invaded his liver. Thank God he called!

After Tom completed the first part of the treatment for E. histo, an ultrasound showed that one of the abscesses in his liver had completely dissolved; another had dissolved by 50 percent, and the third by 20 percent. Another round of treatment followed. The next liver ultrasound showed that all three abscesses had completely dissolved. After this ordeal, Tom did follow-up testing to be certain he had eradicated this infection.

Let's take a closer look at E. histo and other common parasites, and their roles in causing chronic stress.

Entamoeba histolytica

Entamoeba histolytica is one of the most aggressive and invasive parasites on our planet. Five to seven weeks after exposure, it invades nerve and muscle tissue in the large intestine, damaging both and potentially causing inflammatory bowel disease. It can ingest red blood cells, penetrate tissues by boring through their walls, and if it invades the liver, go systemic and travel throughout the body, typically causing dysentery.

As mentioned in Tom's case, E. histo can form amebic abscesses in the liver if not treated in a timely manner. If surgery is performed to remove the abscesses, toxins are released into the bloodstream, overwhelming the body's immune and detoxification capabilities.

E. histo can travel virtually anywhere in the body. It can migrate to the liver, lungs, and even the brain. As a matter of fact, one theory postulates that many appendicitis attacks are caused by E. histo infections. I have noted this correlation several times in my clinical practice.

Blood and stool testing can reliably detect E. histo infections. Treatment necessitates the use of antibiotics and other drugs, as aggressive therapy is required to eradicate this resistant pathogen. A qualified doctor can prepare the body not only for the toxic effects of the medications, but also the toxic load created as the parasites die off.

The liver will be under increased demands from processing the circulating toxins, and healthy bacteria naturally existing in the GI tract will need to be replaced as they are killed off by the antibiotics. The gut will also require nutritional support to help repair and rebuild the blistering and scarring that can occur when a parasite burrows into its lining. And, because the intestinal wall is likely to be damaged from the infection, nutritional supplementation should be employed to aid in mucosal barrier restoration.

Giardia lamblia

Perhaps best known as the organism responsible for "Beaver Fever" or "Backpacker's Diarrhea" because of its proliferation in streams and rivers, Giardia lamblia can completely destroy the surface of the mucosal barrier. As with gluten intolerance, the destruction of the small intestine's barrier causes inflammation, reduction of surface area for nutrient absorption, lactose and sucrose intolerance, and inability to digest fats and oils. It can also result in the formation of deep pockets, in which mucus plugs form, creating an environment that harbors and protects infectious organisms.

Another effect of Giardia infection is hypermotility, in which food moves through the small intestine too quickly and therefore isn't completely digested. The undigested food dumps directly into the large bowel, which creates protein putrefaction and a fertile environment in which yeast, fungus, and other unwanted microorganisms proliferate.

If you ingest Giardia in cyst form, you may have no symptoms. For those with healthy mucosal barrier defenses—recall the prisoner study—the cyst is more likely to be encapsulated and flushed out through the GI tract before it can hatch and replicate. But, if you have compromised mucosal immunity, your body will unlikely be able to eradicate the cyst before it hatches. Within weeks, this cyst can produce millions of Giardia organisms!

Giardia cysts can also infiltrate the gall bladder and enter the ducts through which the liver, pancreas, and gall bladder release digestive chemicals and enzymes into the small intestine. One such duct is the common bile duct, which carries bile from the liver and gall bladder into the small intestine. Infiltration of Giardia cysts into the common bile duct changes the composition and flow of bile and impairs the digestion of fats and oils.

Given the destructive nature of Giardia, you might think that you would have obvious symptoms once infected. This isn't always the case. During the acute phase of an infection, symptoms are apparent, but you might not associate them with a parasitic infection. You might believe that the short-lived diarrhea and fever were caused by flu or bacteria from contaminated food. This point emphasizes the need for routine lab testing to rule out the presence of parasites.

Giardia also produces neurotoxins—toxins that harm the nervous system. These toxins cause depression, sleep disorders, and an inability to concentrate, among other symptoms. Giardia is linked to autoimmune disease, particularly with neurological autoimmune processes such as multiple sclerosis, ALS (Lou Gehrig's disease), and Parkinson's disease. I have found Giardia infections in many of my patients who were chronically ill to the point of disability.

Cryptosporidium parvum

Cryptosporidium parvum is an insidiously invasive organism. Capable of living inside cells, it is so invasive that it can exist in the delicate mucous membranes lining the eyes and the lungs. C. parvum destroys the cells that it inhabits within the gastrointestinal tract, resulting in severe mucosal barrier damage, including inflammation and malabsorption.

Numerous outbreaks of Cryptosporidium throughout the United States have been documented, including one in Milwaukee in 1993 in which more than 400,000 people got acute, watery diarrhea from contaminated municipal water supplies. One hundred and four people died in this incident. One of the challenges presented by Cryptosporidium is that chlorine doesn't destroy it, which makes finding a municipal water supply that is 100 percent free of contamination at all times difficult.

After the acute phase, Cryptosporidium causes intermittent diarrhea or loose stools as it migrates in and out of cells approximately every seven days. Therefore, a classic sign of Cryptosporidium infection is diarrhea or loose stools once every seven to ten days.

Conventional medical doctors steer their treatment decisions with information released in peer-reviewed journals and studies. Sadly, these studies often fail to examine the subtleties of the subjects they engage. C. parvum is a classic example. Most medical doctors will tell you that it does not require treatment. They say it is self-limiting; the body's immune system will kill it. They recommend treatments if the patient's immune system is compromised—often citing cases of elderly patients and patients infected with HIV. I believe this perspective on compromised immunity is absurd.

You don't need to be elderly or stricken with a severe disease to have an immune system incapable of dealing with parasites! A number of my patients have refused my suggestions for taking drug therapies for C. parvum, as we consistently find the bug in stool analysis. Eventually, they accept the fact that they need to get rid of the bug and they are always glad they did.

Because Cryptosporidium is an intracellular parasite, it is difficult to treat. In fact, it was once thought that the only way to kill this parasite was to destroy the healthy cells that it lives in—in other words, kill the host! However, antibiotics proven successful in killing Crypto are now available. I would like to tell you that natural remedies exist for Crypto and other aggressive parasites, but I have yet to see their effectiveness on a consistent basis. However, I don't rule out that there are skilled healthcare providers out there who use effective natural protocols.

Helicobacter pylori

At the beginning of this book, I told a story about a friend who died as the result of an undiagnosed infection. A chronic infection of the bacterium Helicobacter pylori likely caused the stomach cancer that killed him. He was unable to produce adequate hydrochloric acid and couldn't digest his food, particularly proteins. Instead of looking for the underlying cause, he believed he had a hereditary deficiency and that supplementation would replace what was missing.

He was wrong. In fact, the supplements he took only masked the problem. Since he didn't have any of the classic symptoms of an H. pylori infection, such as acid reflux or heartburn, he declined any diagnostic testing. One year after an endoscopy showed a raging infection of H. pylori, he died from stomach cancer.

There was a time when we acquired Helicobacter pylori from

travels in third-world countries. Now we can get it right here in the United States. The statistics on Helicobacter pylori are alarming. An estimated 90 percent of all ulcers are caused by H. pylori infections and almost 50 percent of the world's population may be infected with it. It took years for mainstream doctors to accept that H. pylori is a harmful organism responsible for serious health issues.

The big event that woke up much of the medical community was the awarding of the Nobel Prize for Medicine to Robin Warren and Barry Marshall of Australia in 2005. These researchers were diligent in proving that H. pylori caused ulcers even to the extent of infecting themselves. Their dedicated research earned them the esteemed prize and obliterated the prevailing dogma regarding ulcers.

How does H. pylori cause an ulcer? Because of its shape and the way it moves, the bacteria can penetrate the stomach's protective mucous lining where it produces urease, an enzyme that neutralizes good stomach acids. This weakens the stomach's protective mucus, making stomach cells more susceptible to the damaging influences of certain acids and enzymes, thereby leading to ulcers in the stomach or small intestine.

I recommend stool antigen testing to determine whether you have an H. pylori infection. If you are positive for H. pylori, antibiotic regimens can effectively eradicate the bacteria. Some natural remedies are showing promise as well.

Blastocystis hominis

Listing Blastocystis hominis as a harmful organism may raise a point of disagreement with some in the medical field, but I stand by my conviction that it is a harmful and increasingly common health offender. A lack of clinical research emphatically establishing

"Blasto" as a pathogen—though mounting evidence supports its connection to Irritable Bowel Syndrome—is responsible for the lack of motivation by pharmaceutical interests to develop a drug to target the bug. Mainstream doctors commonly tell their patients that it is "normal" to have this bug in the gastrointestinal tract. My perspective is simple. It is a parasite. It shouldn't be in your body. Whenever my patients were treated for Blasto, their health improved! Its presence in the body is another source of chronic stress that must be removed.

Blasto is a unique, recently discovered microorganism. It was first classified as a harmless yeast in 1912 and later as a protozoan (single-celled organism with a nucleus). As recently as 1998, it was reclassified into its own class, Blastocystea. With this confusion arises the controversy of whether or not Blasto is harmful enough to warrant treatment. Even recent studies validating its damaging effects on the intestinal lining and ability to cause cell death are viewed as inconclusive by many in the medical establishment because of a lack of "corroborating evidence."

I have seen the percentage of my patients testing positive for Blastocystis hominis skyrocket over the past 15 years. I believe we are in the very early phases of awareness about this organism, not to mention the early phases of its epidemic development. Watch for research developments at the Blastocystis Research Foundation based in Oregon (www.bhomcenter.org). I anticipate exciting information from this group that will motivate the healthcare community to take the bug more seriously.

Other Common Parasites

While not as common as the parasites listed above, many other pathogens contribute to the Chronic Stress Response. The following four are the ones I frequently encounter in my patients:

- *Dientamoeba fragilis:* Recent medical literature states that D. fragilis is a harmful parasite causing abdominal pain, bloating, and diarrhea in up to 90 percent of infected individuals. The most common symptoms appear to be intermittent diarrhea and fatigue. In some people, both the organism and related symptoms may persist or reappear indefinitely until appropriate treatment is initiated; multiple treatments may be necessary to eradicate it.

- *Clostridium difficile:* C. difficile is a "bad" bacterium that coexists with good bacteria in our intestines. Fortunately, when you are healthy, the millions of good bacteria keep C. difficile under control. However, taking antibiotics also reduces good bacteria. If your C. difficile population is virile and not killed by the antibiotic, then it can overpopulate your colon, potentially releasing toxins that contribute to colitis. Colitis is a painful irritation of the colon that causes diarrhea and severe cramps.

- *Entamoeba hartmanni:* This parasite is similar to E. histolytica, but does not have an invasive stage and cannot ingest red blood cells. While this makes it less of a danger than E. histo, it still produces classic gastrointestinal symptoms and contributes to chronic stress. It is— like its close relatives Endolimax nana, Iodamoeba butschlii, and Entamoeba nana—considered by many in mainstream medicine not to be problematic in healthy individuals. Again, I believe that scientific research lags in contrast to clinical experience and smart case management.

- *Toxoplasma gondii:* According to the Centers for Disease Control, more than 60 million people in the United States may be infected with the Toxoplasma parasite. As this bug is very common in cats, cat owners are at a high risk of contracting it. While it does not typically cause obvious symptoms, T. gondii can cause brain and eye damage, especially in immunocompromised individuals. Some patients report flu-like symptoms that can be debilitating for up to several weeks. Serum antibody testing must be performed to confirm a T. gondii infection.

Many other microorganisms are responsible for driving the Chronic Stress Response. To address them all would require another book altogether. Just be aware that these bugs are out there—if not inside you—and use common-sense measures to prevent exposure. My family and I utilize annual preventive laboratory testing, and I recommend that my patients do the same. Early identification and treatment of these nasty critters is the best way to prevent their potentially devastating health effects.

Lyme Disease

A discussion on infections would not be complete without mentioning Lyme disease. Lyme is a serious health problem that stirs up debate among health professionals given the controversy over its sources and the complexity of diagnosing and treating it. It may well be the number one emerging infectious disease of the 21st century. It is known to be caused by the Borrelia burgdorferi bacterium, which is transmitted to humans by deer ticks found in woodlands (though evidence is being gathered that supports the notion that humans, mites, mosquitoes, and fleas also transmit the infection).

In many, the first symptom of Lyme is a "bull's-eye" skin rash that forms at the site of the bite. This lesion is red and slowly gets bigger, usually with a clearing in the center. Not all people infected with Lyme notice this type of rash. Infected people may also have flu-like symptoms, such as fatigue, fever, headache, stiff neck, and muscle or joint pain, possibly lasting several weeks. If the early stages of the disease are not recognized and treated, serious problems, such as nervous disorders, heart problems, or joint pain, may develop weeks or even months later.

B. burgdorferi, with its corkscrew shape, burrows into and through the body's tissues. It also travels through the walls of blood vessels. Studies have shown that shortly after infecting a host, the Lyme organism can deeply embed itself inside tendons, muscle, the heart, and the brain. It invades tissue, replicates, and then destroys the host cell as it emerges. Besides causing widespread inflammation through its mode of travel, Borrelia also releases toxins—called bacterial lipoproteins—that trigger many harmful responses.

Lyme disease is referred to as "the Great Imitator" because it resembles other diseases. The fever, muscle aches, and fatigue of Lyme can be easily mistaken for viral infections, such as influenza. Joint pain can be mistaken for arthritis, and neurologic signs can mimic those caused by multiple sclerosis. Conversely, types of arthritis or neurologic diseases can be misdiagnosed as Lyme.

Further adding to the difficulty of diagnosing Lyme is the absence of a standard lab workup. Doctors generally use a variety of different blood tests to accumulate diagnostic data, but the procedures are not consistent given disagreement among doctors. Researchers have developed what they believe to be the best tests for Lyme, but the approval process with the Food and Drug Administration has proven to be arduous. Recently, a great deal of attention has been brought to Lyme's implication as a causative factor in autistic spectrum disorders and Alzheimer's. It is hoped that this will speed up the pace of well-organized research at all levels of science and healthcare.

General information promotes the idea that avoiding Lyme disease is as simple as avoiding tick bites. While the jury is still out on the matter of how Lyme is contracted, I believe that a risk exists to anyone bitten by insects or who has had intimate contact with a Lyme-infected individual. Only time will tell just how severe a health threat Lyme disease represents, but for now it looks like the surface of this problem has barely been scratched. I urge you to become self-educated about Lyme disease and keep your eyes and ears open to news on this emerging epidemic.

Preventing Parasitic Infections

As demonstrated in the prisoner study on Giardia and the mucosal barrier, healthy first-line immunity goes a long way toward preventing infections. As you are now aware, a healthy immune defense relies on good hormone balance and a strong gastrointestinal system. You can take simple precautions daily to help prevent infection.

One of the most effective ways to prevent a parasitic infection is to wash your hands several times throughout the day, especially after contact with people and animals. Make sure you get under the fingernails, and if you bite your fingernails, by all means stop! Antibacterial liquid solutions appear effective for sanitizing on the go.

The vast majority (85 to 90 percent) of reported cases of

food-borne illness in the United States are believed to be caused by a lack of hygiene and food-handling errors in the home and commercial kitchen. Without passing a single new law or hiring any additional government inspectors, food-borne illness could be reduced dramatically if everyone learned simple, safe food-handling and preparation procedures. Many infectious medicine experts recommend peeling and thoroughly washing all fruits and vegetables, thoroughly freezing and cooking meat to kill microorganisms, and avoiding buffets and salad bars that do not appear fresh and well-managed.

If you must eat out, avoid uncooked foods and rare meats, unless you are very confident in the food handlers in the kitchen and dining area. We all love a good meal. However, minutes of satisfaction now are not worth a lifetime of jeopardized health. Be smart and moderate your consumption of high-risk foods, especially in public facilities.

A clean water supply is vital. Drinking bottled water is one option, but some brands—hint: they are better known for their soft drinks—may not be any better than water straight from the tap. In fact, any liquid bottled in a plastic container runs the risk of being tainted by chemicals in the plastic. Water stored in glass or stainless steel is much safer than that stored in plastic, which tends to leech volatile organic compounds in the water. Given that it is unlikely to break like glass or ceramic, stainless steel is my preferred container for liquids. It also seems best suited to preserve the taste.

Water filters are a great option for home and office, especially those that enhance the water after stripping its content (see www.biohealthinfo.com for resources). The minor drawback with all filters is that you need to change and clean them often; otherwise, they become a point of concentration and a breeding ground for the contaminants they're intended to remove. Given the importance of healthful water, the initial setup and ongoing maintenance of a filtration system is worth the cost and effort. And it's not just about the water you drink or cook with. The water you bathe in should also be the purest possible since your skin absorbs it.

Find out what is in your tap water. Contact your local utility and request a copy of the Annual Water Quality Report. This report will give you information about any contaminant violations in your water system and help you decide on a filtration system. Consider the cost savings as well. Bottled water ranges from $0.90 per gallon to $9.00 per gallon. Tap water, on average, costs $0.002 per gallon! Since travelers commonly report picking up parasites, researching your destination before you depart is critical. A good resource for travelers is the Centers for Disease Control website (www.cdc.gov), which provides information on recent outbreaks, necessary preventive measures, and treatment options.

Finally, I cannot overemphasize the risk associated with human and animal contact (conditions caused by cross-contamination between animals and humans are known as zoonotic diseases). Take, for example, my colleague Mike. Early on in our respective clinical practices, Mike did some stool testing, which confirmed a suspected Helicobacter pylori infection. He treated it, and follow-up testing showed successful eradication. Not long after that, familiar H. pylori symptoms such as bloating and acid reflux returned. He tested and again was positive on stool for H. pylori. Since I knew that H. pylori can be transferred by human fluids, I encouraged him to test his wife. His wife, also positive for H. pylori, underwent the treatment alongside Mike.

Months after determining they had been rid of the bacteria, the symptoms returned. Then it came to me: Mike and his wife are dog lovers. They have two big, beautiful Labrador retrievers that they allow to lick their faces, even their mouths! We tested the dogs and, lo and behold, both were positive for H. pylori.

A healthy first-line immune defense and preventive testing of all that we are in physical contact with—human or otherwise—is paramount to preventing chronic stress.

Detecting Parasitic Infections

Unfortunately, no single defining symptom indicates that you have a parasitic infection. Fatigue, night sweats, irregular bowel movements, and stomach irritability are all possible signs of hosting a parasite. However, parasites may not manifest any obvious symptoms or symptoms may be delayed until decades after initial exposure, when the damage is substantial and possibly irreversible.

As mentioned, I recommend that everyone routinely perform diagnostic tests. Stool and blood tests can determine whether you have parasites and identify the type and severity of the infection. Some of my patients delay the collection of their stools or put off getting blood drawn because of the unpleasant nature of these procedures. I have no sympathy for their complaints! A little discomfort is a small price to pay for potentially adding years—and vitality—to your life.

Infectious organism testing is cost-effective and can prevent serious health problems. Skilled microbiologists, who take the time to exhaustively analyze and culture specimens for infectious organisms, can be found in specialty labs like the one I founded, BioHealth Diagnostics.

Getting Rid of the Parasites

Although it's usually best to begin treating parasites as soon as possible, undertaking treatment on your own is not advisable. Using readily available anti-parasitic herbs and "natural" formulas, which are often not strong enough to kill off the parasites, can cause the parasites to migrate deep into the intestinal tissues or other organs, making them more difficult to detect and eradicate. In gluten intolerant individuals, inflammation and deep pockets form in the gut, creating places for parasites to hide and possibly remain safe from both natural products and antibiotics.

Each parasite requires unique intervention. Working with a knowledgeable doctor who is experienced in diagnosing and treating parasites while supporting the body's systems during treatment is imperative. Parasitic infections are one of the greatest threats to your health and chief contributors to the Chronic Stress Response. Be aware; get tested.

Chapter 8

The Mold Effect

Many people—including construction professionals—are either unaware of or in denial about the severe health hazards involved with mold found in buildings. Omnipresent in the environment, molds are one of the two largest groups of fungi, the other being yeasts. High levels of airborne molds in your home, place of work, and other buildings you frequent are a source of chronic stress. Unlike plants, molds lack chlorophyll; they can't produce the food they require from sunshine. Instead, they obtain food directly from decaying organic material, which allows them to thrive in dark, covered areas, outside visual observation.

Common sources of airborne molds include water-damaged walls, foundations, and carpets, as well as contaminated heating, ventilation, and air-conditioning systems. The cellulose in moist building materials such as ceiling tiles, rotting wood, and the paper covering on Sheetrock make perfect substrates for molds to thrive on. Mold seen on metal, glass, or bathroom tile is feeding on an organic deposit from substances such as oils, dirt, or skin cells. Mold can even grow on organic debris trapped within fiberglass insulation. Given a food source, dampness, and an ideal temperature, opportunistic molds can flourish almost anywhere.

Severe examples of building-related illness caused by mold infestations—and related lawsuits—have drawn national media attention. In the last decade, reports of schools, courthouses, and other public buildings being closed for major renovations or demolition because of extensive mold contamination have increased. Significant business, building, and real-estate interests aim to suppress important research and awareness of the dangers of mold to protect the bottom line.

Structures with chronic water or moisture problems are ideal places for mold to thrive. Colonies of mold can proliferate in the damp, dark spaces behind walls, above ceilings, and in aging air ducts. These molds—and the chemicals and toxins they produce— contaminate the air within a building. And beware, not all molds produce the characteristic musty odor. In fact, some produce no odor at all.

Health Effects of Chronic Mold Exposure

The medical community is just beginning to understand the health consequences of chronic mold exposures. For example, the toxins released by an indoor mold called Stachybotrys chartarum are extremely toxic to nerve cells. In addition to being neurotoxins, they suppress the immune system, leading to decreased levels of antibodies and lymphocytes. Stachybotrys, a black and slimy mold, requires an extremely damp environment to proliferate. While spores of wet mold do not easily enter the air, disturbing dry, mold contaminated material can release spores into the air, resulting in the possibility of human exposure.

Other health effects reported by individuals living in moldy homes include recurring cold-like and flu-like symptoms, coughing, chronic bronchitis, sore throat, diarrhea, fever, headache, chronic fatigue, dermatitis, rhinitis, bleeding in the lungs, tightness in the chest, intermittent difficulty in focusing the eyes, neurological symptoms, and general malaise.

In all but the most severe cases of exposure to the most toxic molds, symptoms typically resolve after the source of mold exposure is removed, although the very young and frail have been known to die from such incidents. Even healthy, young people have been known to succumb to Stachybotrys. I recently heard of a man who was remodeling his home. He used an axe to chop into a wall, and unbeknownst to him had unleashed millions of mold spores. The man died from this exposure. Wearing an inexpensive mask could have saved his life.

Mold Case Study: Carol

Carol, a physician and colleague, sought my help with her own case. Carol had not felt well for more than five years. She experienced extreme fatigue, neurological symptoms such as intermittent numbness in her extremities, and a wide array of gastrointestinal symptoms. The parasites C. parvum and H. pylori were recurring infections. She treated these bugs and any other issues we diagnosed, but the problems would return within a short period.

Carol was clearly immunocompromised, but no obvious cause was apparent. I put her on a supplement regimen designed to support and strengthen her immune system. The thought of mold exposure crossed my mind because molds are immune-suppressive, but Carol lived in the desert, where the environment is hot and dry. She repeatedly assured me she didn't have mold exposures in her environment. Carol felt "better" on her supplement program, but most of her symptoms were unresolved. I finally insisted that she run a mold antibodies test to look for an elevated immune response to common indoor molds.

The testing revealed that Carol had severely elevated antibodies to all of the molds on the profile, including Stachybotrys chartarum. I recommended that she call an environmental testing service and instruct the company to test the air in her home and adjacent office. The environmental tests showed dangerously high levels of the molds to which Carol had elevated antibodies.

Carol and her husband relocated while environmental contractors determined the source of the mold in her home and office, and performed the necessary remodeling to remedy the problem. Damaged plumbing was the culprit, setting up the ideal environment for mold to flourish.

To help speed Carol's recovery, I suggested that she purchase a high-quality air filter for her apartment and avoid any dietary sources of mold-loving foods, such as chocolate, mushrooms, cheeses, leftovers, tepid water, fruits and fruit juices (especially citrus), dried fruits, soy sauce, vinegar, and any other foods that may easily become moldy. Inhaled molds, as well as those contained in foods, can colonize in the gastrointestinal and respiratory tracts.

Carol's case verifies how important it is to remove all potential sources of mold exposure. Even so, elevated antibodies to molds can persist for up to a year after the sources of exposure have been removed.

Mold Protection in the Home or Workplace

The process of identifying the location and causes of mold growth is of paramount importance. I urge you to make whatever corrective actions are necessary in your environment. Although this can be an expensive process, it's well worth the price given the potential health consequences.

Particular types of mold release mycotoxins, organic compounds that create toxic reactions in humans. Prolonged exposure to these toxins adversely affects nerve and brain cells. In some cases, such exposure can result in irreversible brain damage and cause problems with eyesight, memory, coordination, balance, and hearing. Mycotoxins are inhaled along with mold spores. Like fungi, molds reproduce by releasing spores into the air, and can therefore be inhaled as mold dust (dried mold).

Another source of irritation from mold exposure comes from substances known as microbial volatile organic compounds (mVOCs). These compounds are produced through fungal metabolism and released directly into the air, often giving off strong or unpleasant odors. Exposure to mVOCs from molds can irritate the eyes and respiratory system and has been linked to symptoms such as headaches, dizziness, fatigue, nasal irritation, and nausea. The effects of mVOCs are not completely understood and research is still in the early stages.

People are exposed to molds every day, usually by touching or breathing them. Because molds naturally exist outdoors and indoors, living in a totally mold-free environment is practically impossible.

As molds grow, spores may be released into the air where they can be easily inhaled. People who inhale large numbers of spores may get sick. Possible health concerns are an important reason to prevent mold growth and to clean up molds in indoor environments.

How can you determine if you might have a mold problem in your home or office? Be on the alert for these signs:
- Buckling floorboards
- Crumbling walls
- Damp basements or crawl spaces
- Discolored areas on bathroom or kitchen tile, caulk, or grout
- Improperly installed siding
- Lack of ventilation (where indoor humidity can accumulate)
- Musty or earthy scents
- Roof or plumbing leaks (especially if undetected for a while)
- Sewer backups
- Unusual stains on walls or ceilings

If you suspect heating and cooling air ducts as sources of mold in your home, hire contractors to clean or replace them. Carpets are another potential substrate for molds, especially in homes built on cement slabs. The concrete "sweats" and moisture is absorbed into the carpeting, creating an ideal environment for molds. To properly install carpet over a concrete floor, the concrete should be covered with a plastic sheet, which is then covered with plywood sub-flooring for insulation. Even carpets made of synthetic fibers trap all kinds of organic material on which molds can feed. Never install carpet in areas that have high potential for water contact, such as kitchens or bathrooms.

While mold spores can never be eliminated from the indoor environment, the way to control indoor mold is to control moisture.

Follow these tips:
- Be sure your home has adequate ventilation. Use exhaust

fans in the kitchen and bathroom that vent outside your home. Also make sure that the clothes dryer vents outside your home.

- Clean up molds when you find them and eliminate the related sources of moisture. Use enzyme-based products for safety and effectiveness.
- Fix any leaks in roofs, walls, or plumbing in your home to eliminate a source of moisture for mold.
- Keep the humidity level in your home between 40 percent and 60 percent. Use an air conditioner or a dehumidifier during humid months and in damp spaces, such as basements.
- Make every attempt to clean up and dry out your home thoroughly and quickly (within 24 to 48 hours) after any type of flooding.
- Periodically clean bathrooms with mold-killing products, being careful to avoid skin contact or inhalation.
- Remove and replace carpets and upholstery that have been soaked and cannot be dried promptly. Avoid using carpet in rooms that tend to be moist, such as bathrooms or basements.
- Replace absorbent materials such as carpeting, ceiling tiles, and Sheetrock if they become moldy and can't be thoroughly cleaned.

In areas receiving a lot of rain, basements can flood from the hydrostatic pressure of underground streams. The best solution for this appears to be installing French drains around the foundation. French drains let water in but channel it into a pit, where a pump removes it from the basement and pumps it out and away from the structure. A friend who builds homes told me that a natural but often impractical solution to a leaky basement is to plant a willow tree near the house where the basement leaks. The willow tree's demand for water decreases the hydrostatic pressure.

Mold problems in public buildings such as schools can sometimes be attributed to construction practices employed for energy efficiency. These buildings are tightly sealed in an attempt to maximize the efficiency of heating and cooling systems. Poor ventilation impedes moisture from escaping, causing mold growth and creating what has come to be known as "sick building syndrome."

People working in these buildings are not only exposed to molds, they're also exposed to chemicals that outgas from modern building materials. Be aware of the likelihood of mold in public buildings. If you or your children spend a lot of time in them, ask questions of the people responsible for construction decisions and be persistent until you get solid answers.

Concerned? Get Tested!

Are mold exposures a significant source of chronic stress for you? Ask your doctor to test your blood for antibodies to common indoor molds. Also test the air in your home and urge that testing be performed in any public buildings you frequent. Home testing kits can be purchased inexpensively (see www.biohealthinfo.com for resources). The samples can be sent to a professional environmental analysis company to analyze and confirm your mold problem.

Not all members of a household will have obvious symptoms from mold exposures. Those with a genetically predisposed sensitivity, or other significant sources of chronic stress, may become symptomatic while other members of their family remain healthy. Sensitive individuals warn of potentially hazardous exposures for all.

Chapter 9

Heavy Metal Toxicity

Heavy metal exposure can wreak havoc on your health. Time and time again, I have seen profound health improvements after the removal of metals from patients. Metals can bind to cellular sites normally occupied by essential minerals, disrupting metabolic activity. They inhibit the uptake of calcium, depriving bone tissue of essential nutrition and potentially causing osteoporosis. Metals can also damage the body's natural antioxidants, leaving you more susceptible to oxidative stress. Vague and puzzling symptoms are sometimes related to toxic levels of heavy metals.

From my observation, the biggest offenders are mercury, nickel, lead, cadmium, arsenic, and aluminum. These elements are called "heavy" metals because they are comprised of large atoms with high atomic weights. A number of other metals can be harmful to your health, such as platinum, barium, tin, beryllium, and even high levels of chromium and copper.

I will focus on the sources and consequences of the main culprits. The lists of potential sources are not necessarily comprehensive, and safe alternatives may exist. I urge you to be aware of your environment and be vigilant for potential toxic exposures.

Mercury

This discussion begins with mercury because so many people have been exposed to it through amalgam dental fillings. One of the most prevalent causes of chronic illness I've encountered is from the mercury and silver comprising these fillings. The American Dental Association perpetuates the untruth that amalgam dental fillings (made from approximately 50 percent mercury) are safe. However, the mercury in fillings has caused innumerable illnesses, degenerative diseases, and deaths.

Despite volumes of research indicating otherwise, the ADA maintains that mercury, when mixed with silver to create amalgam dental fillings, becomes inert and is therefore harmless. In reality, mercury in filling materials releases toxic gas into your mouth and through tissues. This organization continues to turn its back on science at immeasurable cost in human pain and suffering. Financial interests and the status quo overwhelm rational thought and concern for public safety. If you have metal fillings, I urge you to get them removed by a biological dentist who can refill them with safe composite materials.

For centuries, mercury has been known as one of the most poisonous substances on earth. Hippocrates, the father of modern medicine, remarked on its toxicity more than 2,000 years ago. Despite its known dangers, mercury has been used in industrial processes and medications for over 1,000 years, causing degenerative disease and neurological damage. In fact, the expression "mad as a hatter" described people poisoned by mercury from working in hat factories.

Besides dentistry and occupational settings where elemental mercury is used, most of the health risk from mercury exposure is due to methylmercury from fish consumption. Mackerel, shark, shellfish, and swordfish top this list. Tuna may also contain methylmercury, but usually in smaller amounts. Adults who consume a large quantity of these fish on a regular basis are at a high risk for toxicity.

Other common sources of mercury exposure include:
- Batteries
- Broken fluorescent light bulbs
- Chlorine bleach
- Grains and seeds treated with methylmercury to kill bacteria and fungi
- Latex paints
- Pesticides and fungicides
- Plastics
- Printer's ink
- Vaccines

Mercury is uniquely dangerous because it is a liquid at room temperature and vaporizes easily. This is why you shouldn't attempt to vacuum up a mercury spill from a broken thermometer unless the vacuum's exhaust system is vented to the outside. Mercury is absorbed upon skin contact, inhaled into the lungs, and seeps through the intestines when ingested.

Mercury toxicity may be associated with hundreds of symptoms and conditions. The most common include depression, neurological damage, emotional instability, mood swings, inability to concentrate, sleep disturbances, irritability, abnormal heartbeat, pressure and pain in the chest, high or low blood pressure, and anemia.

Nickel

Nickel is toxic to the body in all but trace amounts—the body needs minute amounts to maintain strong immune function. However, nickel is responsible for more allergic reactions than all other metals combined, and it can have a negative impact on the immune system. Nickel toxicity depletes the body's zinc stores, because nickel substitutes for zinc in important metabolic pathways that support immune function. This happens because nickel and zinc are approximate in size, weight, and positive charge. But that's where the similarity ends.

Nickel is so toxic that it's used to promote cancerous tumor growth in laboratory rats. Studies show that occupational exposure to nickel dust at refineries results in increased incidences of pulmonary and nasal cancer. Several of my patients have had cancers possibly linked to nickel toxicity. Stainless steel braces and bridges leech nickel into the oral cavity, contributing to the development of tumors. In fact, a registered nurse I knew died of cancer believed to have been a result of the nickel in her stainless steel braces that caused tumors to grow in her mouth and neck.

Unbelievably, like mercury, the use of nickel in dental appliances has been declared safe by the ADA.

Nickel toxicity can contribute to a wide array of symptoms and conditions, including, but not limited to food allergies, inflammatory bowel disease, Crohn's disease, ulcers, colitis, nausea, diarrhea, compromised digestion and immunity, cancer, lupus, arthritis, chronic fatigue, capillary damage, cognitive problems, muscle tremors, paralysis, malaise, insomnia, endometriosis, and cirrhosis of the liver.

Gerard Mullin, MD, PhD, a gastroenterologist with Johns Hopkins University and one of the country's leading Crohn's disease researchers, states that nickel—as well as other metals—is a primary source of stress to the immune system, including the depletion of zinc and dysfunction of the mucosal barrier.

Most exposures to nickel are dental, dietary, or industrial. Common sources include:

- Auto exhaust
- Batteries
- Buckwheat, cabbage, herring, hydrogenated oils, legumes, kelp, oats, and oysters (nickel-containing foods can aggravate an existing toxicity)
- Cookware
- Cosmetics
- Dental bridges and root canals
- Fertilizers
- Industrial emissions
- Jewelry
- Nickel-plated alloys
- Pens
- Tobacco smoke

Nickel is used as a catalyst in the hydrogenation of vegetable oils, including corn oil, peanut oil, and cottonseed oil, as well as margarine. Grains may be stone-ground, but if stainless steel is used to grind them, the nickel in the stainless steel can contaminate the grains. Stainless-steel cookware can transfer some nickel to foods; acidic foods in particular can leech nickel from stainless steel. Frequent handling of coins, especially—you guessed it—nickels, is another source. While there are many ways to be exposed, those at the highest risk are workers in the metallurgy fields who are constantly exposed to metal dust and debris.

Lead

I'm sure you've heard the expression "Get the lead out." Well, that's not a bad idea. Lead is a poisonous element that targets protoplasm, the living substance inside your body's cells. Lead has a particular affinity for the cells of the nervous system, including the brain, spinal cord, and peripheral nervous tissue. It can even infiltrate bone, weakening skeletal structure. Lead exposure can increase blood pressure and cause fertility problems, nerve disorders, muscle and joint pain, irritability, and memory or concentration problems.

Lead toxicity can contribute to a wide array of symptoms and conditions, including, but limited to:

- Cirrhosis of the liver, hair loss, birth defects, heart problems, thyroid dysfunction, and kidney disease
- Frequent colds and infections of all types
- Muscle weakness and muscle pain
- Nausea, vomiting, diarrhea, constipation, abdominal pain, loss of appetite, and weight loss
- Seizures, learning disabilities, headaches, tremors, dizziness, depression, fatigue, malaise, nervousness, disorientation, hyperactivity in children, nerve damage to hands and feet, loss of sight, and mental retardation

By far the greatest source of concern is lead paint found in much of our nation's older housing and the fact that young children often inhale or make oral contact with surfaces painted with it. Until 1978, lead paint was commonly used in construction. Today, the U.S.

Department of Housing and Urban Development (HUD) estimates that about 38 million homes in the United States still contain some lead paint.

Generally, adults develop lead poisoning as the result of an occupational exposure or hobby. Occupations related to house painting, welding, renovation and remodeling, and the manufacture and disposal of ammunition and car batteries carry a particularly high risk of lead exposure. Workers in these occupations must also take care not to leave their work sites with lead-contaminated clothing and tools, or with unwashed hands and facial hair, lest they spread lead to their vehicles, homes, and ultimately to friends and family members.

Common sources of lead exposure include:
- Batteries
- Body powders
- Candle wicks
- Henna (hair and skin dye)
- Imported canned food
- Paint chips and dust
- Pesticides
- Plastics
- Tap water (contaminated by soldered joints on copper pipes)

Cadmium

Cadmium is an extremely toxic metal commonly found in industrial workplaces, particularly where ore is processed or smelted. Buildup of cadmium levels in water, air, and soil occurs in industrial areas where safeguards are inadequate. Cigarettes are another source of cadmium exposure. Although there is generally less cadmium in tobacco than in certain foods, the lungs absorb cadmium more efficiently than the digestive system.

What happens when you are exposed to cadmium? Cadmium tends to accumulate until a threshold of resistance is surpassed. Once this occurs, high blood pressure, which promotes hypertension, often develops. Some individuals with high blood pressure have blood cadmium levels three to four times higher than those with normal blood pressure.

In addition, like nickel, cadmium can replace zinc in critical metabolic pathways, impairing immune system function. Increased exposures to cadmium damages the liver and kidneys, softens bone, and even causes a loss of sense of smell.

Cadmium exposure is associated with the following symptoms and conditions:

- Abdominal pain, weight loss, vomiting
- Disrupted iron, copper, and magnesium metabolism
- Immune suppression, immune dysfunction, slow healing
- Sodium retention, low body temperature
- Sore joints, acne, anemia, decreased fertility, lung disease

Common sources of cadmium exposure include:

- Batteries
- Cigarette smoke
- Dental amalgam fillings
- Fertilizers
- Film development processes
- Fish from polluted water
- Incinerated by-products of rubber and plastics

- Metal plating
- Paints
- Particles from auto tires and brakes
- Silver polish

Arsenic

Arsenic is a naturally occurring element found in the environment, especially in food and water. However, exposure to high levels of the inorganic form, such as that found in wood preservatives, insecticides, and weed killers, can be deadly. Known for its role in poisonings, arsenic can be inhaled or ingested, or, to a lesser degree, absorbed through the skin. Arsenic targets the central nervous system, causing convulsions and death. As little as one-tenth of a gram accumulated over a two-month period can produce death, and arsenic is carcinogenic at much lower levels.

Studies have linked long-term arsenic exposure in drinking water to cancer of the bladder, lungs, skin, kidney, nasal passages, liver, and prostate, according to the U.S. Environmental Protection Agency. It is also associated with cardiovascular, pulmonary, immunologic, neurological, and endocrine problems.

Arsenic can enter the water supply from natural deposits in the earth or from industrial and agricultural pollution. It is used for a variety of purposes within industry and agriculture, and is a byproduct of copper smelting, mining, and coal burning. Industries in the United States release thousands of pounds of arsenic into the environment every year.

Arsenic toxicity can contribute to a wide array of symptoms and conditions, including, but not limited to:

- Cardiac disease, lung disease, diabetes, and diseases of

the blood vessels
- Damage to the liver and kidneys (causing jaundice and fluid loss or fluid retention)
- Difficulty healing from injury
- Electrolyte imbalances or depletion
- Fever
- Hair loss
- Hyperpigmentation (darkening) of the skin and vitiligo (white patches)
- Increased risk for cancer of the bladder, lung, kidney, liver, and colon, and prostate
- Iodine and folic acid deficiencies that damage the thyroid (resulting in goiters)
- Skin problems, including skin cancer

Common sources of arsenic exposure include:
- Fungicides, herbicides, insecticides, and pesticides
- Paints
- Seafood
- Water (polluted by runoff from pesticides, natural mineral deposits, industrial disposal)
- Wood preservatives

Shellfish in particular can accumulate arsenic—an organic form called arsenobetaine that is less harmful—and should be eaten selectively and sparingly or avoided completely.

Aluminum

Aluminum is an environmentally abundant element to which we are all exposed. Although it is considered a "light" metal compared with other heavy metals because of its low atomic weight, it still causes serious health problems in those exposed to unsafe levels. Inhaling aluminum is one of the more harmful exposures, because this transports the metal through nerves in the nose directly to the brain.

Workers who inhale aluminum dust may have lung problems, from coughing to chronic emphysema. Some workers who breathe aluminum dust or fumes showed decreased performance in tests that measure nervous system function. People with kidney disease typically store excess aluminum in their bodies, increasing the risk of developing bone or brain diseases.

Some studies suggest that aluminum is linked to Alzheimer's disease—a condition in which cognitive function and memory diminish over time, eventually leading to senility and dementia. The cognitive function of Alzheimer's patients is reported to improve when aluminum is removed from the body with desferroxamine, a chelating agent. Chelating agents are used to bind metals and remove them from the body.

Aluminum exposure may be associated with the following symptoms and conditions:
- Alzheimer's disease, cognitive difficulties, headaches
- Bone loss, muscle aches, physical weakness
- Higher susceptibility to colds and flu
- Severe dryness of the mucous membranes and skin

Common sources of aluminum include:
- Aluminum cans, paints, silicates, and spray paints
- Antiperspirants, deodorants, and shampoo
- Automobile exhaust
- Baking powder
- Buffered aspirin
- Cat litter

- Cigarette filters and smoke
- Cookware
- Food additives
- Lipstick
- Medications

One study documented that the concentration of aluminum in water heated in an aluminum coffee pot is increased by 75 times. The use of aluminum cookware is probably the most common source of exposure in daily life, despite public awareness of the problem.

Diagnosing Heavy Metal Toxicity

Heavy metals can accumulate in the body over time. If one's health progressively deteriorates, most doctors are unlikely to consider heavy metals as a cause, and low levels of metal toxicity are difficult to diagnose. Long-term, low-level exposures, in which the toxic load gradually increases, represent a dangerous source of chronic stress. On the other hand, acute exposures to heavy metals, while potentially deadly, are often easier to identify and treat.

As an investigation into your Chronic Stress Response evolves, it is wise to have your doctor run tests that can detect levels of heavy metals. Excellent lab testing is available using urine, hair, feces, and blood. Each medium has its own respective value in the diagnosis and monitoring of detoxification. Lab tests not only identify levels of metals, they can also correlate immune system dysfunction with specific metal exposures (see www.biohealthinfo.com for resources).

Chelation and Detoxification

If tests confirm that you have heavy metal toxicity, your doctor should develop a detoxification program to remove the metals, while using care to not overwhelm your immune and detoxification systems. Heavy metal detoxification should be conducted under the guidance of a doctor experienced in the proper use of chelation, saunas, and other treatments that aid in the safe removal of heavy metals. My patients, both children and adults, who have tested positive for heavy metal toxicity have all responded very well to carefully managed detoxification programs.

People with heavy metal toxicity commonly have chemical toxicity as well—and the reverse is true. This is why it's important to remember that the process of liberating chemicals from the body will invariably liberate heavy metals. Again, it takes special knowledge and experience to safely and effectively administer heavy metal and chemical detoxification.

In more acute cases where larger amounts of metals are ingested, vomiting may be induced. Washing out the stomach (gastric lavage) may also be useful. You may require intravenous fluids for complications from poisoning, such as shock, anemia, and kidney failure. Like many of the stresses discussed in this book, treatment measures depend on the severity and timing of the exposure.

I would be remiss not to mention the link between heavy metals and autistic spectrum disorders. Experts in the treatment of these disorders routinely share success stories with me about children with autism who improved as a result of undergoing heavy metal removal through chelation. There is evidence—though aggressively repressed by interests linked to the pharmaceutical titans—that some childhood vaccinations contain toxic preservatives that contribute to autism, attention deficit disorder, and related disorders. It saddens me greatly when I see money taking priority over the general welfare of human beings, especially children.

Regardless of age or symptoms, discover whether you are harboring toxins. With any chronic illness, heavy metal toxicity must be considered, particularly if you have metal in your mouth or a history of risky exposures. Toxicity from a single heavy metal can cause the Chronic Stress Response.

Chapter 10

Chemically Stressed?

Given my history of environmental illness and the chemical exposures that set the stage for it, this topic is near and dear to me. Had I known earlier in my life that I was being chronically exposed to chemicals, I could have consulted a specialist for testing and treatment and possibly have avoided years of suffering. I not only developed multiple chemical sensitivities—to the extent that I was forced to live in remote rural areas in sterile rooms—but the Chronic Stress Response unraveled my overall health.

There are two types of chemical exposure: acute and chronic. Acute exposures, such as burns from a corrosive cleansing agent or inhalation of high levels of pesticides, are obvious, and typically result in unmistakable symptoms very quickly. Chronic exposures, on the other hand, can be very subtle or go unnoticed, with few or no apparent symptoms. The latter form poses a menacing source of chronic stress.

Take the effect of chemicals on hormone (endocrine) function, for example. An endocrine disruptor is a synthetic chemical that, when absorbed, either mimics or blocks hormones, disrupting the body's normal functions. This disruption can happen by altering normal hormone levels, suppressing or stimulating the production of hormones, or changing the way hormones travel through the body. Endocrine disruptors can enter air and water as a by-product of manufacturing processes, and by burning plastics and other materials. Studies have found that endocrine disruptors can leach out of plastics, even the type of plastic used to make intravenous bags for hospitals!

We're exposed to a multitude of chemicals in our air, food, water, and common consumer products. We are often unaware of exposure to these potentially deadly elements because we can't see or smell them. Notable exceptions are smog, exhaust, and pollution from factory smokestacks. Each year in the United States alone, several million reported poisonings occur from accidental and intentional exposure to toxic products used in the home. However, we know this number is much greater, because toxic exposures that don't cause immediate symptoms generally go unreported.

The pervasive nature and harmful effects of chemicals cannot be ignored. The United States alone produces about 400 billion pounds of synthetic chemicals annually. That's approximately 80 pounds of chemicals a year for each person on the planet. About 55,000 chemical compounds are in production and the Environmental Protection Agency officially lists 48,000 chemicals. Of these, fewer than 1,000 have been tested for toxic side effects and only about 500 for adverse health effects.

Common sources of chronic chemical exposure include:

- Alcohols and glycols (such as antifreeze and ink/ paint solvents)
- Aldehydes, ethers, esters, and ketones (formaldehyde being the most common)
- Aromatic compounds (most notably benzene, toluene, ethylbenzene, and xylenes) found in groundwater, soil, and fuels
- Artificial detergents
- Colognes
- Drugs (therapeutic and recreational)
- Food additives (such as aspartame and sulfites)
- Gases (fumes and air pollutants such as industrial ventilation and smog)
- Halides; also called halogens (found in water supplies; these include chlorine, fluorine, bromine, and iodine)
- Nitrogen (petrochemical by-products)
- Paints and solvents
- Pesticides

Our behavior as a society suggests that we don't recognize the inherent health risks that chemicals pose. Are we complacent because we feel helpless to alleviate such an overwhelming problem? Are we addicted to the perceived lifestyle benefits that chemicals provide? Is corporate America intent on reaping profits from lucrative chemical sales without regard for the cost to society, including human suffering?

Chemically Exposed: Two Examples

The Hobbyist: Neal came to me for help with reversing his chronic fatigue, depression, and poor mental function. I inquired about his work and home environments in an attempt to determine possible exposures to various chemicals and heavy metals. Although he didn't report any chemical exposures that would suggest high levels of toxins, his lab tests revealed such evidence. When I called to discuss my findings with him, his wife answered the phone. She said her husband was shopping for supplies for his hobby—building and painting fiberglass boats. Neal hadn't reported this hobby to me. I also discovered that he did his work in a barn and, because of the cold climate, the windows were closed most of the time.

Resins used in fiberglass construction and paint contain numerous toxins. Breathing these fumes is hazardous, especially when they are concentrated in a room with poor ventilation. Upon learning about his hobby, I contacted Neil and recommended that he immediately stop his boat project until we resolved his health problems.

About one year later, Neil regained his health. He was able to continue his hobby by keeping the windows open, using fans to exhaust dangerous fumes and by wearing protective gear. This case ended happily because we identified the cause of his health complaints and treated them before irreversible consequences developed.

Not Just for War Veterans: I have treated and have witnessed the disabilities of several Vietnam veterans who were exposed to Agent Orange. Dioxin, the active ingredient in Agent Orange, causes slow and severe damage to the brain and nervous system. One man couldn't walk down a hallway without bumping into the walls. He would stumble and fall, and then, with great effort, would pick himself up, only to bounce off the walls and stumble and fall again. His was one of the saddest cases I have ever witnessed.

You don't have to fight a war in a third-world country to be exposed to dioxin. A by-product of industrial discharges, dioxin is one of the most potent carcinogens known to man. Environmental dioxin exposures are related to industrial discharges and the burning of wastes. Discharges from polyvinyl chloride (PVC) and pesticide production plants—as well as the waste from garbage incinerators, pulp mills, and backyard burn barrels—release dioxin fumes into the atmosphere.

Dioxin was one of the toxic chemicals found at Love Canal in Niagara Falls, New York. On August 2, 1978, the New York State Department of Health declared a state of emergency at Love Canal when it became clear that the 20,000 tons of chemical waste disposed there from 1920 to 1953 were the cause of the startling increase in cases of cancer, birth defects, and miscarriage rates among local residents.

We must all be aware of our surroundings to prevent or eliminate exposure to toxic chemicals. The Love Canal case, on the other hand, demonstrates how we are victims of the reckless poisoning of our planet by industrial powers. Both of the previous examples describe fairly obvious exposures. Unfortunately, most chemical exposures are not so obvious.

Something in the Air

Chemicals are omnipresent. They spew from industrial smokestacks, engine exhausts, burn sites, and other modes of waste release, rising into the atmosphere, then falling back to earth as acid rain onto the soil, where plants absorb them. These plants become our food and the food for the animals we eat. Residual toxicity from breathing and eating creeps into our bodies and does damage, typically without obvious signs. Do I recommend that you stop breathing and eating? Of course not. However, you should be aware of exposure risks and should not ignorantly let chemical stress steal your health.

Many of us are exposed to contaminated air every day. Perhaps the most common and insidious source for most Americans is exhaust from motor vehicles. Car exhaust has been known to aggravate respiratory conditions, increase the severity of allergies, exacerbate depression, adversely affect immune system function, and even trigger heart attacks.

The risks associated with chemicals from vehicle exhaust are well documented. A study by the American Thoracic Society proves that living near major traffic zones is a sure way to increase the chances of serious illness. The study, performed in 2005 in San Diego, found that children living within 75 meters of a major road had an almost 50 percent greater risk of having had asthma symptoms in the past year than did children who lived more than 300 meters away.

The largest national study of a specific population and air pollution was published in 2006. The study suggests that elevations in fine particulate air pollution increase cardiovascular and respiratory hospitalizations across the United States. Researchers at Johns Hopkins and Yale universities monitored 11.5 million Medicare enrollees in 204 urban counties between 1999 and 2003. They found that short-term spikes in particulate-matter pollution—including soot, dust, smoke, and liquid droplets—resulted in a greater percentage of people being hospitalized for heart and lung ailments, obstructive pulmonary disease, respiratory infections, and peripheral vascular disease than when the air was cleaner.

You don't need to be outside to be exposed to chemicals. Safety indeed begins at home. According to the Environmental Protection Agency, indoor levels of air pollutants can be two to five times higher—and occasionally even 100 times higher—than outdoor levels. Consumer products and building materials are largely responsible. Plywood and particle board, as well as certain materials used in curtains, carpets, and furniture, release formaldehyde fumes and other aldehydes. Adhesives, solvents, shoe polish, and artificial degreasers and air fresheners are all sources of pollution. Some people even store fuels, pesticides, and toxic household cleaning products indoors!

The air in your home needs to move. If toxic gases or particulates are in a stagnant environment, they will stay there, possibly saturating carpets and furniture. Highly sophisticated air filtration equipment is available to help keep your air clean, whether in your home, office, or car. Natural, environmentally safe air fresheners and cleaning agents can replace the chemically loaded products that bombard us in advertisements. Safer alternatives to chemically treated carpets, drapes, paints, furniture—and virtually all household items—are available.

Eat, Drink, and Be Wary

Food: A major source of chemical exposure is the pesticides that have invaded our food chain. Soils become tainted through acid rain, thus exposing plants and animals. Even "certified organic" foods may contain some levels of chemicals. Despite this, they are still strongly preferred to the chemically treated foods that are not certified organic. The risk of eating or drinking contaminated products is largely tied into the origin of the food. Some areas of the country are notoriously high in contaminated water and soils, while others are relatively free of pollutants.

Since few of us enjoy the rare freedom to grow and raise our own foods in a pristine environment, the general rule of thumb is to raise your consciousness and practice some common sense when choosing what to put into your mouth.

Rule #1: Don't eat fast food. Besides the fact that it lacks the nutrient levels of healthfully prepared foods, the meats in fast foods are laden with growth hormones, the vegetables are laced with pesticides, the soft drinks are loaded with refined sugar and artificial flavors, and fast foods too numerous to mention have had their color and taste modified by manufactured chemicals. And yes, these points are also true about foods that you can't "drive through" to acquire.

Rule #2: Read the ingredients on labels and use common sense! In many situations, thanks to the required ingredient lists on foods and drinks, you have the power to decide whether you will be exposed to chemicals in food and drinks. However, this is not always the case when eating out or visiting the bar for a cocktail. Ask your server or bartender about the specific contents of the meal or drink. They are obligated to provide you with the facts. Avoid artificial sweeteners (such as aspartame and saccharin) and coloring agents, as well as high fructose corn syrup; these are not foods, they are poisons.

Water: The EPA estimates that volatile organic compounds (VOCs) are present in one-fifth of the nation's water supplies. VOCs are emitted as gases from certain solids or liquids. They can enter groundwater from a variety of sources. Benzene, for example, may enter groundwater from gasoline or oil spills on the ground surface or from leaking underground fuel tanks. Other examples of commonly detected VOCs are dichloromethane (methylene chloride), an industrial solvent; trichloroethylene, used in septic system cleaners; and tetrachloroethylene, used in the dry-cleaning industry.

VOCs vary considerably in their harmful effects. Researchers have collected an extensive amount of information about the health effects of VOCs, from animal studies and from studies of human exposure to large quantities of chemicals in the workplace. Safe drinking water levels called health risk limits (HRLs) have been established for many VOCs. HRLs are levels of chemicals in drinking water considered safe for people to drink, including sensitive people such as the very young or the elderly. I would not rule out, however, that lobbyists for chemical manufacturers influence these levels. Does it seem possible that financial interests would influence public health in a negative way? Of course!

VOCs at levels higher than the HRLs are harmful to the central nervous system, the kidneys, and the liver. VOCs may also cause irritation when they contact the skin, or may irritate mucous membranes if inhaled. Some VOCs are known or suspected carcinogens. For VOCs that do not cause cancer, conservative methods are used to establish HRLs at levels considered safe, even if the water is used every day for drinking, cooking, bathing, and laundry.

For carcinogens, HRLs are established so that drinking water with levels above the HRL will cause no more than one additional person to get cancer for every 100,000 persons exposed over a lifetime of use, a relatively small risk according to the ones at state and federal agencies who write the rules. Water containing chemicals at levels lower than the HRLs is considered safe to drink. However, individuals who find their water contains chemical contaminants at low levels should choose to stop drinking their water and investigate treatment options.

Your exposure to these chemicals depends entirely on where you are and how much local water you drink. Many of us would like to think that the bottled water we drink is safer, even healthier, than the water that runs from our taps. Yet bottled water—even purified water—is not necessarily completely free of contaminants;

it simply has to test below FDA and state-allowed levels of certain contaminants.

In 2005, the ABC news program 20/20 sent five different national brands of bottled water and one sample of tap water taken from a New York City drinking fountain to a lab for testing. The results showed no difference, in terms of unhealthful contaminants, between the bottled waters and the tap water. I believe that filtering your own tap water is the most healthful and economical option. It also spares the environment from pollution caused by the manufacturing and disposal of the plastic bottles that carry the water.

Filtration is the key to minimizing exposure. Since contamination in drinking water is invisible to the naked eye and varies from bottle to bottle and spout to spout, the more treatments you apply—such as reverse osmosis and carbon filtration—the better.

Water is an amazing substance. No living thing can survive without it. Although we drink it, wash and swim in it, and cook with it, we tend to overlook the special relationship it has with our lives. Droughts cause famines and floods, bringing death and disease. Water makes up over half of our body mass and without it, we die within a few days. Water is the second most common substance in the universe (behind hydrogen) and fundamental to star formation. Life cannot evolve or continue without liquid water, which is why there is so much interest in finding it on Mars and other planets and moons. That water plays a central role in many of the world's religions is unsurprising. Appreciate this amazing substance, be vigilant, and make your food and drink choices based on intelligent awareness. Take nothing for granted.

Plastics

The widespread use of plastics represents a source of exposure to chemicals. Plastics are omnipresent in our society, particularly in homes, work environments, hospitals, and schools. Many common household items are made from plastics, including baby feeding bottles and teething toys, kitchen appliances, cables, and floorings. Plastics contain plasticizers, which are chemicals—and known carcinogens—called phthalates that give products their flexibility. They get into our food and water from packaging and containers and, because they're volatile (readily vaporized), they also exist in the air we breathe.

In fact, the often admired "new car smell" comes from the out-gassing of plasticizers! About the time you smell them, these toxic chemicals have likely made their way through your lungs into your bloodstream and are headed for your brain and internal organs. The damage is typically subtle—contributing not to overt symptoms, but to the Chronic Stress Response.

Consider some guidelines to avoid common exposures to plasticizers:

- Buy meat from a butcher and have it wrapped in paper.
- Do not defrost foods in their packaging materials.
- If you buy cheese or any other fatty food wrapped in plastic, cut off the outer layer in case plasticizers are leaching into the food.
- Try to avoid plastic containers whenever possible. Despite popular myths about certain types of plastics being better than others (depicted by the imprinted recycling codes, known as Resin IDs), there is no substantiation to be found. Whenever possible, use stainless steel or glass to

contain your foods or drinks.
- In the kitchen, use glass containers or ceramic cookware.
- For your pet, use glass or ceramic food and water bowls.
- Never microwave food in containers such as margarine tubs, cottage cheese cartons, or deli containers. I also recommend that you do not use microwaves at all.
- Try to find natural substitutes for plastic products. For example, instead of plastic bags for your groceries, use paper or cloth bags.

Chemically Induced Oxidative Stress

Exposure to chemicals accelerates oxidative stress. Oxidative stress is what occurs when your molecules interact with foreign substances—such as chemicals—and electrons are displaced. This creates an electrically charged, unstable molecule, known as a free radical. It actively seeks to become stable by interacting with the nearest available molecule. Having no prejudices, it targets proteins, fats, and even DNA.

Many things cause oxidative stress, including excessive exercise and vitamin deficiency, but nothing promotes its acceleration and resulting damage like toxic exposures. In simple terms, free radicals can harm or destroy healthy cells. There are everyday examples of oxidative stress, such as when an apple browns or iron rusts. But these nuisances don't compare to what unstable molecules can do inside your body.

Your primary defense against free radical damage is a complex group of chemical reactions involving your body's sulfhydryl group defense. A sulfhydryl group is a sulfur atom combined with a hydrogen atom. Sulfhydryl groups are effective in removing poisons and toxins from the body. They have the ability to neutralize free radicals by binding with their unpaired electron, rendering the free radical chemical compound nonreactive.

Foods with a large amount of the amino acid cysteine can significantly help support the sulfhydryl groups. High levels of cysteine are found in onions, garlic, chives, red pepper, egg yolks, asparagus, dry beans, soybeans, sesame seeds, pumpkin seeds, and sunflower seeds.

Oxidative stress can be minimized with the intake of antioxidants in the diet. Foods known to be high in antioxidants are green tea, colorful fruits, and green vegetables (especially kale and spinach). You can also supplement your diet with therapeutic levels of antioxidants like coenzyme Q10 and alpha lipoic acid. A diagnostic test marker called Lipid Peroxides, typically done inexpensively on a urine sample, can measure your body's oxidative stress load.

Multiple Chemical Sensitivities

My doctor and mentor at Henrotin Hospital's Environmentally Controlled Unit, Dr. Theron Randolph, spoke of chemical overload as analogous to water in a rain barrel. The buildup of chemicals in the body is similar to rain filling a barrel. There's a threshold beyond which the barrel can't hold any more water and overflows.

Similarly, our bodies get to the point where they can't handle even a minor exposure to chemicals. At that point, we meet our individual thresholds of reactivity; we become overburdened and our "rain barrel" begins to overflow. People experience sensitivities to things that may have been only annoyances in the past: vehicle emissions, cologne, paint fumes, and cigarettes. For example, instead of the inhalation of secondhand cigarette smoke being merely bothersome, it might trigger a terrible headache and neck pain.

A simple and relatively reliable indicator of chemical toxicity is an increased sensitivity to light. If you always feel the need to wear sunglasses, even when it is not very sunny, you may have a problem with chemical overload. Sensitivity to sound is also a clue. If you can't tolerate even a radio playing softly in the background, you may be experiencing chemical sensitivity.

Commonly referred to as multiple chemical sensitivities, I experienced the state of experiencing symptoms to virtually all chemical exposures, as described in the introduction.

Detoxification and Recovery

If laboratory testing reveals chemicals, your doctor must develop a detoxification program to remove them, while taking care not to overwhelm your immune and detoxification systems. Chemical detoxification—like heavy metal detoxification—should be conducted under the guidance of a doctor experienced in the proper use of chelation, saunas, and other treatments to aid in safe detoxification.

As previously noted, people with chemical toxicity commonly have heavy metal toxicity as well—and the reverse is true. The process of liberating chemicals from the body will invariably liberate heavy metals. Again, special knowledge and experience are needed to put someone through heavy metal and chemical detoxification safely and effectively.

Far infrared saunas are an effective and relaxing means of assisting detoxification. When I went through my 30-day dry-heat sauna program, the gentler far infrared saunas had not yet been developed. Nevertheless, the dry-heat sweating saved my life, because as long as I had poisons in my system, I had no chance at recovery.

You must minimize or eliminate the sources causing Chronic Stress Response to escape chronic illness. Although chemical stress may seem unavoidable because of its omnipresence, it is critical that society at large does everything in its power to enforce controls and limits on the use and disposal of toxic chemicals. Personal as well as governmental and industry awareness and action are essential.

Chapter 11

Electromagnetic Radiation

The old Invisible Man television series featured a character that could not be seen. He could sneak up on anyone and get away with just about anything. There was no warning that he was present. The same is true of electromagnetic and radioactive energy fields—we generally have no indication that they are present.

With the ever-increasing reliance on electronic technologies, few places remain where you can escape the energy of satellite signals, wireless Internet connections, cellular phones, computers, and other modern technologies. By living in cities, we are constantly bombarded by energy from these devices. And even rural residents are exposed daily to the myriad of electrical fields produced by their household appliances. Can you imagine what it would look like if you could see every radio frequency, every microwave transmission, and every satellite signal? It would be quite a psychedelic light show!

Dr. William G. Timmins

Until about 100 years ago, the only radiation to which humans were exposed came from natural sources, predominantly sunlight. With the advent of electricity, man-made sources of electromagnetic fields and radiation have increased our exposure exponentially. Electromagnetic waves are produced by the motion of electrically charged particles. These waves are also called electromagnetic radiation, because they radiate from the electrically charged particles. They travel through empty space as well as through air and other substances, including the human body.

How Does Radiation Affect Your Body?

Electromagnetic radiation assumes the form of waves in space. An important characteristic of electromagnetic waves is their frequency, which is related to how much energy they carry. High-energy/high-frequency electromagnetic waves have a short wavelength, while low-energy/low-frequency electromagnetic waves have longer wavelengths. While the entire range exerts some influence over your body's energy, the shorter the wavelength, the more destructive the effect.

High-energy radiation such as X-rays and gamma rays are known as sources of ionizing radiation. Nonionizing, low-energy radiation has a longer wavelength and includes everything from ultraviolet (UV) rays to microwaves. Ionizing radiation is potentially damaging to the DNA of your cells. That sources of ionizing radiation such as X-rays and gamma rays are harmful to cells has been known for some time. Increasing evidence is mounting that sufficient long-term exposure to nonionizing radiation can also destroy cells and set up cancerous conditions.

More than 30 international studies on electromagnetic radiation have found conclusive links to cancers. In a school in San Francisco, 22 cases of cancer occurred among staff working in the front of the school. No cancer was found in those working in the back. Large electrical transformers were located at the front of the school. Similar results have been documented in Colorado, Sweden, and Manhattan Beach, near Los Angeles. As a result, in Sweden, high-power transmission lines are now buried in insulated piping with counterbalancing EMFs (electromagnetic fields).

Alternating current (AC), which has a frequency of 60 hertz (cycles per second), is very low-energy electromagnetic radiation. For a long time, the electromagnetic fields produced by this current were considered harmless. However, today, growing concern exists that long-term exposure to even low-energy electromagnetic fields can cause cellular damage. For example, a recent study by the University of Los Angeles found that leakage of AC through the heart by electromedical devices results in heart racing and fibrillations.

Though uncommon, I have even seen patients suffer from immediate nausea, headaches, and weakness when exposed to common electronic devices such as televisions and stereos. Each person has his or her own degree of sensitivity to this invisible stress. For those already in a prolonged Chronic Stress Response, the effects are bound to be more acute, given an already weakened disposition.

The following are several examples of what electromagnetic radiation is doing to humans:

- A growing number of people living near high-voltage power lines are developing life-threatening illnesses.
- Some have taken their local power companies to court, claiming the companies had information on the harmful health effects of EMFs for years, but deliberately withheld

that information from their customers.
- Electric utility workers with high exposure to magnetic fields had more than twice the risk of brain cancer than workers with lower exposures.
- Of 35 international research studies on EMFs, 33 have made a conclusive link between brain tumors, leukemia, and other forms of cancer.
- Women in electrical occupations have a greater chance of dying of breast cancer than those working in nonelectrical occupations.
- Women who use video display screens that emit strong electromagnetic fields are at greater risk of miscarriages than women using low-field video display screens.
- Workers with moderate to high exposure to electromagnetic radiation were three to four times as likely to develop degenerative brain disease, such as Alzheimer's disease, compared with workers who did not work around strong electromagnetic fields.

A Tale of EMF Ignorance

I once met a man who was fighting leukemia. He came from a small northern California town with a population under 600 and an exceptionally high cancer rate, particularly of leukemia, the blood cancer. I learned from him that his town was situated in a ravine over which a power company had installed many high-tension power lines and transformers.

This man told me that, at the time, there was a lot of controversy over this matter. Politicians and medical authorities never acknowledged that the power lines had anything to do with the residents dying from cancer. I knew that it was an invisible source of chronic stress, compromising the core functional systems of this town's residents. Sadly, no one in authority was willing to investigate the relationship between the presence of high-tension power lines and abnormally high cancer rates.

Speculation from "experts" suggested that many of the cancer-related deaths resulted from exposure to pesticides, chemicals, some common infectious agent, or possibly a virus. No one dared suggest that this sudden onset of deaths could have been the result of the high-tension wires and the strong electromagnetic frequencies they emitted. Although this man believed his leukemia was a direct result of the power lines, he did not survive to make his case.

EMFs as Life-saving Treatments

There is another side to EMFs. During my first 10 years in clinical practice, I was interested in learning about advances in the treatment of cancer, so I visited cancer clinics throughout the United States and Mexico. Although I became familiar with both mainstream and alternative therapies common in the United States, the therapies being used in Mexico caught my attention. Without restrictions imposed upon them by the American "cancer industry," Mexican clinics are able to evaluate and use new therapies from around the world.

Many Saturdays, I'd donate my time at a clinic in Tijuana. One morning, while I ate breakfast at a restaurant, a tall, thin man in his fifties asked if he could sit with me because there were no empty tables. I welcomed him to join me. As he sat down, I couldn't help noticing the grapefruit-sized tumor growing on the right side of his neck.

When I asked him about it, he told me the doctor who diagnosed his malignant tumor in the United States said it was too large to be treated surgically and that his cancer was fatal. That motivated him to search for alternative therapies. Instead of repeating the same dire prognosis, the Mexican doctors predicted it would take about 10 days to dissolve the tumor and that whatever was left over would pass through his bowels.

I've always been skeptical of promises of miracle cures. I believed that his Mexican doctors had infused the man with false hope. However, knowing the stress this man must have been under—and not wanting to dash his hope—I wished him well.

Two weeks later, I ran into him in the same restaurant and I was amazed to see that the tumor had totally disappeared! He told me that on the tenth day of treatment, he saw what was left of his tumor pass in a bowel movement, just like the doctors had told him it would. I was happy for him—and intrigued. Obviously, the treatment was effective, but I wanted more than anecdotal evidence; I wanted to know how this oddly wonderful event had occurred.

The man was eager to recount his treatment. He told me that the principal therapy his doctors used was surgical implantation of an electrical probe directly into the tumor. An electromagnetic field then pulsed through this probe into the tumor, causing it to dissolve little by little. On the tenth day, the tumor had completely disappeared. I never saw this man again and often wonder if the disappearance of his tumor truly meant that he was in remission.

Fascinated by the use of energy healing in the form of electromagnetic energy to destroy a tumor, I was motivated to learn as much as I could about this type of therapy and, conversely, the ability of electromagnetic fields and radiation to cause cancer. Subsequently, I met numerous people in Mexico who were trying to beat cancer using electromagnetic therapy; some survived and some did not. Most had this in common: they had received a terminal diagnosis and had come to Mexico, where healing innovations were not restricted.

Detection Is Protection

I had a patient who realized that his years of insomnia had begun when he started sleeping in his bedroom, having previously fallen asleep at his desk and having spent the night on the day bed in his study for several years. To satisfy his wife's desire to have her husband sleeping by her side, he began going to bed after he finished reading. This is when the insomnia began. It wasn't until 12 sleepless years later that he made the connection that something in his bedroom was keeping him up at night, and it wasn't his wife's snoring!

What did he do? He checked his home with an electromagnetic field detector, called a Gauss meter, and found an extremely high electromagnetic field coming from a fuse box located behind his refrigerator in the kitchen. The kitchen and bedroom shared a common wall and the head of their bed sat right up against this wall. When he moved the bed to the opposite side of the room, he began to sleep deeply and through the night. Perhaps other issues were at play, but taking this simple step immediately relieved his insomnia. Apparently, electromagnetic fields were a chronic stress for him and could have been implicated in his insomnia, depression, chronic fatigue, and other associated health problems.

A Gauss meter should be an essential investment for anyone intent on reducing physical stress. It will quickly identify the risks associated with frequented locations, especially home and work exposures that are taken for granted as being "safe." Effective Gauss meters for personal use can be purchased from between $50 to $500, depending on range of detection and features.

Prevention and Therapy

Here are some of the many ways you can minimize your exposure to electromagnetic fields. Some people, depending on their existing health status, will be more affected by radiation than others. Nevertheless, we should all be aware and protect our children and others who cannot make their own decisions (see www.biohealthinfo.com for resources).

- Avoid unnecessary X-rays. For example, obtain copies of previous X-rays when you change from one dentist or doctor to another. Often, there is no need to take new X-rays.
- Have an electric radio/alarm clock on your nightstand? Get rid of it. You are exposing your head to radiation while you sleep.
- Electromagnetic shielding is available for common household appliances, and certain types of transmitters can counterbalance electromagnetic fields in most buildings.
- Get radiation shields for your cellular phone and other wireless devices. Minimally, go hands-free with your phone to keep the device at a distance. Cellular phones and other wireless communication devices bombard you with electromagnetic radiation. In my opinion, common sense dictates that a device transmitting satellite signals should not be near your body! Much of the evidence

pointing to cell phone radiation is inconclusive, suggestive, or construed as circumstantial. However, this is because it is difficult and even unethical to perform testing on humans, and is unpopular with the communications industry, which aims to suppress any research that could harm their bottom line. I predict that the cell phone industry will eventually resemble the tobacco industry, paying out billions of dollars to mop up a mess of deception.

- If you are prone to muscle weakness in particular areas of your body, be suspicious of seemingly benign sources of radiation such as digital watches, portable music players, etc.
- If you must use a microwave oven—a device that promotes malnutrition—keep your distance while it operates. These devices are radioactive.
- If you sleep on a heated waterbed, unplug the heater and put a thick, insulating pad between the water mattress and the sheet. Of course, the best solution would be to replace the heated waterbed with a more conventional mattress. Beware of mattresses with motors. Pressing a button to adjust your bed may seem like a great idea, but you are sleeping on a hotbed of radiation, even when the motor is off.
- Keep computers, monitors, and related peripherals away from your head, because long-term microwave exposure is a suspected source of cancer.
- Nearly every household appliance, especially those with an electric motor, produces electromagnetic fields. Since the energy from electromagnetic fields drops off markedly

as you move farther away from the current generating them, you can minimize exposure by moving away from electric appliances while they are in operation. Use a Gauss meter to determine a safe distance to be from a particular electrical appliance while it's in use.

- Replace electric blankets with thick quilts or down comforters.
- Replace fluorescent light bulbs with full-spectrum bulbs.
- Shave with a blade or a battery-operated razor instead of one that needs to be plugged into an outlet.
- Televisions generate electromagnetic fields even when not in use, from the remote control reception for powering on and off. If possible, unplug your TV when it's not in use and place it at least 10 feet from your bed.
- Use low- radiation computer monitors.
- Wear a research-backed pendant or bracelet that helps neutralize electromagnetic fields.

In addition to avoiding exposure whenever possible, the use of certain herbs and nutrients such as iodine, vitamins A and C, zinc, rutin, grape seed abstract, quercetin, and pycnogenol are recommended to protect and detoxify your body—especially your thyroid gland, which is particularly vulnerable to the effects of radiation exposure. Also, two key actions—enhancing your immune system by adopting healthy lifestyle factors and minimizing or eliminating chronic stress—will help prevent compromised hormone, immune, digestive, and detoxification system function.

Additional remedies are available. Homeopathic therapies use subtle energy frequencies that help tune the body's energy. Acupuncture, massage, bodywork, osteopathy, and chiropractic are hands-on therapies that can help. Acupuncture, which has been a part of traditional Chinese medical practice for over 5,000 years, is based on an understanding of the energy fields that naturally run through the body, and has been a decisive factor for successful health outcomes in many of my chronically ill patients. Your body is alive thanks to energy, so why allow harmful energy to come near you?

Electromagnetic radiation is pervasive and inescapable. However, my intention is not to scare you into living in a remote cave! The message here is simple: be conscious. Do not expose yourself to potential sources of stress if you don't have to. Of course, this is the message throughout this book: avoid all sources of stress that drive the Chronic Stress Response.

Natural Radiation from the Earth

Another source of radiation comes from the earth's own energy grids and subterranean influences. The most prevalent sources of this radiation are Curry/Hartmann global grid lines and black streams. Commonly referred to as geopathic stress, this natural source of radiation can influence health in negative ways, but you will be hard pressed to find healthcare providers, even in the so-called alternative field, that do not discount the concept of earth radiation as sheer quackery or pseudo-medicine. I like to investigate all possible sources of chronic stress, regardless of their acceptance in conventional healthcare and their predominance in public awareness.

I have heard from some patients, "We have felt uncomfortable ever since we moved into this house; our health has deteriorated and our previously happy family has become miserable." Have you ever wondered why you felt uneasy when you walked into a particular room? You may have low energy, or you may not sleep well. Electromagnetic fields interfere with the movement of oxygen and water at a molecular level. The actual effects depend on the individual's general health status, how strong the lines are, how much electricity is traveling on them, how wide they are, and their intensity.

Curry/Hartmann lines. Different energy fields, mainly the Curry and Hartmann fields, neatly divide the earth into grids. The Curry lines, named after their discoverer Manfred Curry (a Swiss physician) in the 1950s, run –45 degrees and 45 degrees of north, forming a grid where each square is about 12 feet. The lines themselves are said to be about 4 inches wide. The Hartmann lines, named after the German physician Ernst Hartmann, are about 2 inches wide and are separated by about 5 feet. A node is the intersection of these perpendicular lines, and is the area of highest radiation. Special meters and dowsing instruments can detect the locations of these nodes.

Black streams. These can be defined as underground water veins or streams that give off radiations that may be harmful to life above them. Harmful radiation rises in a vertical plane from the underground stream to the earth's surface and above. Black streams intersecting with Curry or Hartmann fields greatly intensify the level of radiation.

Much can be done to ameliorate or remove geopathic stress. To shield a residence from the effects of geopathic stress, traditional Chinese devices include the building of a "Dragon Wall" (a screen wall with an undulating ridge) or digging a carefully placed ditch. Modern Western methods include carefully placing crystals, copper coils, and radionic devices, all of which can alter energy frequencies.

I have addressed the two predominant sources of geopathic

stress. There are others, and I urge you to learn about them. It is a rather fascinating topic, whether or not related to health. While you may be scoffed at by your healthcare provider for considering such matters, do not be discouraged. Learn and decide for yourself if it makes sense that there is more to this planet than dirt! If you suspect that your home, and particularly your bed, could be in the crosshairs of geophysical radiation, seek the aid of someone experienced in detecting and ameliorating the source.

Chapter 12

Trauma, Inflammation, and Pain

The effects of trauma, inflammation, and pain must be understood by anyone seeking to minimize the Chronic Stress Response.

Trauma is defined as an injury caused to living tissue from an extrinsic agent. Physical trauma can result from injuries such as falls, cuts, burns, and anything else that damages tissues. Inflammation is the body's natural response to heal damaged tissues. When physical trauma causes chronic inflammation, critical physiological functions become increasingly compromised. As a result, the body has a tougher time coping with the inflammation and pain that compromised these systems in the first place.

Significant traumas—especially long-lasting ones—increase the production of cortisol, the primary anti-inflammatory hormone, and can result in Adrenal Syndrome. As discussed in Chapter 4, chronic stresses such as inflammation cause hyperstimulation and exhaustion of the adrenal glands from demands on cortisol production. Add trauma to a body with exhausted adrenals and now you have a destructive cycle, with the adrenal glands becoming more fatigued and the body less capable of resolving its inflammation and pain.

Let's consider whiplash, a physical trauma that induces severe pain and inflammation. A common whiplash injury occurs when the driver of one vehicle collides with the rear of another vehicle. The driver who was rear-ended receives a whiplash injury. Because of tissue and possible skeletal damage, the whiplash inflames the discs, muscles, and ligaments supporting the vertebrae of the neck. It also causes head trauma and accompanying inflammation, because the brain literally gets bounced around inside the skull upon impact.

The inflammatory cascade to the neck that results from a whiplash injury stimulates the production of cortisol and can ultimately lead to Adrenal Syndrome. A whiplash injury can also have a harmful effect on the vagus nerve, which transmits signals from the brain to the gastrointestinal tract, heart, and larynx. Often, people without digestive issues develop gastrointestinal symptoms and disorders after experiencing a whiplash injury. The resulting digestive maladies then become another source of chronic stress, further increasing the total stress load on the body.

Inflammation is a localized, protective response that occurs in the body as the direct result of an injury or the destruction of tissues. Inflammation is actually an immune response intended to destroy, dilute, or sequester the injured tissue, as well as any infectious agents that might be causing tissue damage. Inflammation involves a complex series of events designed to protect the rest of the body from the by-products of the damage that has occurred in a localized area and brings healing to the injured area.

In its visible, tactile, acute form—such as when you hit your thumb with a hammer—inflammation appears red, hot, and swollen. Inflammation is obviously painful and can cause loss of function. Low-grade, chronic inflammation, such as the inflammation that might occur in the small intestine of someone who is gluten intolerant, might not be painful or perceptible at all. However, subclinical inflammatory processes—such as those associated with gluten intolerance—are a serious problem and a major source of chronic stress, handicapping the healing process.

Inflammation is a complex process that can be either beneficial or damaging to the body. Inflammation can be a response to gross tissue damage induced by some form of trauma. Inflammation is also one of the body's first responses to infections as the body tries to rush immune cells to the affected tissue to defend against infection. These types of inflammation are beneficial to the body because they aid in destroying the pathogen and help in the healing process. The body may also trigger inflammation in an area with no threat or foreign invader, indicating the previously discussed autoimmune condition in which the body perceives its own tissues as foreign.

Pain is an unpleasant sensory experience associated with tissue damage. We've all experienced the mild pain of a minor cut, burn, or muscle strain. However, pain resulting from a shattered bone, serious burn, ruptured spinal disc, or cancer can persist 24 hours a day, seven days a week, and become a source of intense chronic stress. Many people consider inflammation and pain as a part of everyday life, something they must deal with as natural to the aging process. I disagree. Inflammation and pain are not normal at any age, and the failure to address them can lead to a disruption of critical physiological systems. Tissue swelling caused by the inflammatory process is one of the primary reasons we experience pain.

Chronic pain commonly disrupts sleep. Sometimes such pain is so disruptive that you can't get the rest necessary to recover from the trauma causing the pain. Without sufficient rest and recovery, your adrenal hormone reserves become depleted. This further exacerbates the state of Adrenal Syndrome that began with the initial physical trauma and related inflammation and pain.

Pain Control

Chronic pain is difficult to treat clinically and yet, if you have chronic pain, addressing it as soon as possible is crucial, ideally using a method that has no toxic side effects. Unless your pain cycle can be broken, recovery from the original trauma may be impossible because your body gets stuck in the Chronic Stress Response, handicapping the healing process.

Depending on its severity and location, numerous therapies are available for dealing with pain. They include:

- Acupuncture
- Chiropractic
- Cold and heat applications
- Energetic therapies like biofeedback, breathwork, hypnosis, and Reiki
- Exercise regimens designed to strengthen injured areas
- Homeopathy
- Massage
- Osteopathy
- Over-the-counter products like ibuprofen or acetaminophen (for short-term use only)
- Physical therapies such as whirlpools and thermal treatments

- Prescription drugs such as hydrocodone (Vicodin) or prednisone (as a last resort or when the pain is absolutely unbearable)
- Rest and relaxation

Integrative Rehabilitation

The single most important factor in developing a treatment plan for pain is to first accurately diagnose its cause, and then create a comprehensive, integrated rehabilitation program. As mentioned in the first chapter, I once worked in drug and alcohol intervention and rehabilitation with my brother, Bob Timmins, the founder of the Adolescent Substance Abuse Program. I administered biofeedback to adolescents enrolled in stress management programs, as well as adult patients in the chronic pain unit. Initially, I was reluctant to accept this position because I had no prior experience working with patients with chronic pain. However, when I realized that many of them were being treated with narcotics like morphine, I felt compelled to develop treatments that would help minimize their use of these addictive, toxic drugs while still providing effective pain relief.

We used various methods including biofeedback, visual imagery, muscle tensing, and relaxation, and breathing techniques. I worked with each patient to identify which of their senses they favored to enhance their ability to participate in the treatments. Some people are visual learners, others auditory or kinesthetic. Once we learned their preferred modes of learning, I was able to create personalized pain-control techniques. To my surprise and delight, the methods were quite successful. In many cases, these techniques helped patients significantly reduce or eliminate their need for pain medications.

In treating inflammation and pain, doctors should select an approach that best meets the needs of the patient and has the fewest side effects. Most medications have toxic side effects that impose their own stress on the body. These should be avoided or limited whenever feasible. It really comes down to one's tolerance for pain. Certain pain "killers" like morphine and hydrocodone can be highly addictive, thus becoming a chronic source of stress if used over time. In some cases, pain medications and anti-inflammatory prescription drugs may be the only viable option, especially when crisis intervention is necessary. However, over time they can become less effective and, worse yet, may undermine critical bodily functions.

The cumulative effect of toxic medications can damage the liver; sometimes this damage is irreversible. While certain drugs may be highly effective at alleviating the sensation of pain, they can actually impede the healing of the initial trauma by being a contributing source of stress on the liver and other organs, and by inhibiting the healing aspects of the inflammatory response.

In the interest of patients' recovery and long-term health, doctors should modify their treatments to minimize the use of harmful drugs as soon as the pain becomes tolerable. During the course of "stepping down" their medications, physicians can introduce nontoxic therapies to take the edge off the transition.

A Study in Pain: Paula

A colleague of mine made the clinical observation that many of his patients with serious degenerative diseases had experienced head trauma, often very early in life. The correlation between head trauma and degenerative disease seemed like a stretch to me, so I categorized his theory as just that: an interesting theory. I didn't think much about this again until I was treating Paula, a 36-year-old woman who was completely disabled as a result of chronic fatigue, fibromyalgia, depression, anxiety, insomnia, loss of appetite, short-term memory loss, and poor cognitive function.

Because of Paula's memory and cognitive problems, I suspected that a head injury may be causing her illness. However, Paula was unable to remember any event involving significant head trauma. With her consent, I contacted her parents to determine whether they could recall such an incident.

In speaking with them, I learned about two major head traumas. Paula had been dropped on her head by a nurse shortly after being born. And, when she was four months old, she fell backwards in her highchair, hitting her head on a hard floor. She spent the next six months in a coma. Paula's parents felt so guilty about the incident that they never discussed it with her.

When I learned about these events, I began to wonder whether my colleague could have been correct about the correlation between head trauma early in life and chronic illness later in life. Could the head trauma 36 years earlier be the cause of Paula's chronic illness?

It is possible that Paula's symptoms were related to chronic stress caused by head trauma and its effect on critical systems of her body when she was a baby. As with all degenerative illnesses, Paula's health problems didn't happen overnight. They were the result of cumulative stress that undermined her health over time. That the injuries she sustained as an infant set the stage for poor health is possible, making her more vulnerable to other health issues than most children and young adults. When I learned of her early history of head trauma, I decided to use the same treatment regimen that I would apply to someone with a concussion.

As part of her treatment, Paula received extensive bodywork and biofeedback to retrain her neural pathways and reestablish healthy control mechanisms linking her brain and critical body systems. After several months of treatment, Paula regained her mental, emotional, and physical health. Eventually, she was able to return to work full time and care for her family.

I believe that my colleague was on to something.

As you can see, physical trauma and its related pain and inflammation can be significant sources of chronic stress. When we are able to heal from inflammation and pain, the chronic stress cycle is broken, the exhausted adrenals are repaired, and the body regains its balance.

PART III

The Four Lifestyle Factors

Laura, a patient, came to see me while enduring major situational stress. She was fatigued, depressed, and not sleeping well. As we discussed her personal life, she made it clear she could not (or would not) do anything to change her stress level. She believed she had no other response available to her. She also made it clear that she had very little money and did not want to do any laboratory testing or purchase nutritional supplements. I knew I could help her if she was willing to change the negative perception and internalization of her stress; however, she was not receptive.

Alternatively, I explained that to better handle her stress, she needed to be absolutely disciplined about maintaining a regimen of healthy diet, exercise, and sleep. She agreed that she could do those things and followed my suggestions. Within three or four months, her depression and fatigue lifted and she was sleeping much better, despite her ongoing situational stress.

Laura was able to cope with the stress because she had addressed three critical lifestyle areas: nutrition, sleep, and exercise. Removing commonly offensive foods—like those containing dairy and gluten—along with practicing eating habits that help stabilize blood sugar levels, went a long way in stabilizing her brain chemistry, thus stabilizing her moods.

The Power of Choice

There is no denying that we are all born with genetic predispositions, both strong and weak. However, additional factors are required for our vulnerabilities to manifest in health problems. Many of us tend to hide behind the illusion that we can get away with reckless living and, when the resulting illness strikes, run to a doctor to relieve the condition. In reality, there is rarely adequate time to reverse the damage caused by years of poor lifestyle decisions. The Chronic Stress Response may be unstoppable once core functional systems have been permanently impaired.

Poor lifestyle choices are generally a matter of choice and the number one precipitating factors in causing our genetic predispositions to manifest as sickness and disease. In fact, poor diet, inadequate sleep, lack of exercise, and mismanagement of mental and emotional stress contribute to ill health more than any other single factor.

Fortunately, you have the power to improve your health and longevity by making choices that support a healthier lifestyle. Implementing small and consistent changes in how you live in the present can prevent illness and disease for years to come. This chapter briefly covers the four principle lifestyle habits that support your foundation for optimal health. They are diet, sleep, exercise, and stress management. While each habit could easily fill a thick book, I will attempt to distill what I believe are the most fundamental points.

Eating to Thrive

Many well-publicized "diets" claim to be the best and the healthiest. Personally, I believe an optimal diet exists for each individual, based on his or her unique biochemistry. There may be a popular diet out there that works for you, but most likely you'll need to refine the guidelines to suit your unique needs. Working with a skilled nutritionist, developing and trusting your intuition, listening to your body, and maintaining day-to-day discipline will help you dial in an eating plan that satisfies your taste buds and meets your body's nutritional requirements.

Blood Sugar Balance. Regardless of the diet you follow, the primary goal should always be the same: maintaining good blood sugar (glucose) control. You can achieve and maintain optimal health only when you are on a diet that promotes hormone balance; that balance depends on a steady blood sugar level. Eating the proper combination of proteins, fats, and carbohydrates regularly and in moderate amounts helps to sustain that balance.

Blood sugar control occurs when insulin and glucagon, two hormones produced by the pancreas, are in balance. Carbohydrate consumption and the resulting rise in blood sugar induce the stimulation of insulin, the hormone responsible for lowering blood sugar and storing excess blood sugar as fat. Protein consumption induces the stimulation of glucagon, the hormone that promotes the mobilization and utilization of fat for energy and, in the process, raises blood sugar.

Insulin and glucagon are antagonists, meaning that the secretion of one acts to balance or modulate the effects of the other. Above-average levels of insulin caused by a diet high in sugar, processed foods, and unhealthy fats is associated with almost every disease known to humankind, especially cancer, diabetes, and cardiovascular disease.

Signs of low blood sugar consist of headaches, brain fog, shakiness, fatigue, worry, carbohydrate cravings, and lethargy. Signs of high blood sugar consist of anxiety, racing mind, nervous energy, headache, difficulty thinking and concentrating, and cravings for protein or fat.

If your blood sugar is too low, you will mobilize cortisol to break down muscle, organ, and bone tissue—not fat—to ensure that a constant supply of blood sugar is delivered to your brain and the rest of your body. In effect, your body digests itself to continue operating. If your blood sugar is sustained at high levels, metabolism becomes chaotic and blood vessels may become damaged, which in turn creates a cascade of undesirable events. Stable blood sugar levels, on the other hand, form a strong foundation for hormone balance and homeostasis.

Glycemic Index. You can ensure that you're eating glycemically balanced meals by becoming familiar with the glycemic index (GI) and glycemic load (GL) of the foods you eat. The glycemic index is a number that refers to the rate at which a particular food causes glucose levels to rise in the blood. The more rapidly a food converts to blood sugar, the more insulin your body makes and the harder it is to maintain good blood sugar control.

As a general rule, all above-ground vegetables—such as broccoli, lettuce, and cabbage—have a low glycemic index (less than 55). All below-ground or root vegetables—such as potatoes, carrots, and yams—have a higher glycemic index (greater than 70). Corn chips, instant rice, rice cakes, bagels, white and whole wheat breads, watermelon, and dried dates are other examples of carbohydrates with high glycemic indices. Most whole grains and whole raw fruits have a moderate GI (56 to 69). However, the more processed these foods are, the higher their GI. For example, whole wheat has a glycemic index of 40 compared with whole wheat flour, which has a GI of 73.

A glycemically balanced meal includes larger amounts of low-GI carbohydrates (above-ground vegetables) and smaller amounts from moderate- and high-GI carbohydrates (below-ground vegetables and grains). Along with your carbohydrate choices, you must include protein to balance the level of insulin to glucagon, as discussed above. When choosing the proportion of carbohydrate to protein, always consider the carbohydrate's glycemic index.

If a carbohydrate has a high glycemic index, eat about one portion of carbohydrate to one portion of protein. Let's say you want eggs and potatoes for breakfast. Because potatoes have a high glycemic index, you should eat roughly the same amount (by weight in grams or by portion size) of eggs as you do potatoes. However, if you scrap the potatoes in favor of carbohydrates with a lower glycemic index—such as green peppers, onions, and mushrooms—you can increase your portion of carbohydrates by two or three times that of the eggs (your protein).

Glycemic Load. The glycemic index doesn't tell us how many carbohydrates are in a serving of a specific food. This is why Glycemic Load (GL) can be more useful. Glycemic load takes into account the glycemic index of a food and the amount of carbohydrates in a typical serving of that food. As an example, let's compare carrots to white pasta.

Fifty grams of carrot carbohydrate has a glycemic index of 131, and 50 grams of pasta carbohydrate has a glycemic index of 71. On the surface, carrots look like an undesirable food that will raise our blood sugar faster than white pasta. However, a serving of one whole carrot contains only 4 grams of carbohydrate. A one cup serving of pasta has 40 grams of carbohydrate. This means that the GL, which adjusts for serving size, is much lower for carrots.

A serving of carrots has a glycemic load of 5.2. The glycemic load of one cup of pasta is much higher, at 28. To have the same glycemic load from carrots, you would have to eat nearly two pounds! This shows how the glycemic index can be misleading. When eating a normal serving size, a food with a high glycemic index will not necessarily raise blood sugar quickly.

The formula for calculating GL is straightforward: multiply the GI value of a food by the amount of carbohydrate per serving, less the fiber, and divide the result by 100.

The formula for calculating glycemic load (GL)

GL = (GI x carbohydrates less fiber) / 100

The examples below are based on GL ranges of low, moderate, and high

Low GL < 10   Moderate GL 10–14   High GL > 15

Example of a high-GI/low-GL food

A 120-gram serving of watermelon has a GI of 72 and the available carbohydrate is 6 grams (the amount of fiber contained in this serving does not warrant inclusion in the calculation). Therefore, the GL of watermelon is (72 x 6) / 100 = 4.3.

Example of a low-GI/high-GL food

A 180-gram serving of cooked whole wheat spaghetti has a GI of 37. The amount of available carbohydrate is 36 grams (42 grams of carbohydrate minus the approximate 6 grams of fiber content). Therefore, the GL of whole wheat spaghetti is:

$$(37 \times 36) / 100 = 13$$

As you can see from the examples, a high-glycemic index food may have a low-glycemic load. However, a low-glycemic food may have detrimental effects because of its high-glycemic load. Therefore, you don't need to avoid all high-GI foods, but do control how much you consume at any one time.

Keep in mind that individual dietary requirements vary, depending on a person's genetic make-up, activity level, and age. When creating a balanced meal, a general rule of thumb is to have approximately three times the amount (in volume, not weight) of low-GI to high-GI vegetables or grains. Books and online references listing the glycemic indices and glycemic loads of common foods are readily available.

Optimally, you'll experiment to determine your ideal ratio of carbohydrates, proteins, and fats for each meal and snacks. It may take creativity, awareness, and persistence, but the payoff will be greater health and vitality. In general, if you feel mentally and physically alert throughout the day, and are not hungry for four or more hours after a meal, this is a good sign that you're eating frequently enough and in the right balance. Your body sends signals when you're out of balance—e.g., fatigue, brain fog, carbohydrate cravings, or anxiety. Don't ignore them!

Choosing the Right Proteins. When choosing your proteins, consider these two criteria:

- A complete versus incomplete protein.
- Low fat versus high fat, as well as good fat versus bad fat.

A complete protein contains all of the essential amino acids that the body must obtain through food each day, preferably at each meal. These amino acids are called essential because they are necessary for life and the body cannot manufacture them. All animal products, except gelatin, contain complete proteins. All vegetables, grains, nuts, seeds, and most legumes are incomplete proteins and must be combined to create a complete protein.

Low-fat sources of protein include most fish, the white meat of chicken and turkey, lean pork, veal, most legumes, and low-fat dairy products. Because these proteins are less dense, they generally can be consumed in greater quantity per meal and more frequently.

High-fat protein sources include red meats, duck, the dark meat of chicken and turkey, halibut, mackerel, swordfish, eggs, whole milk dairy products, nut butters, nuts, and seeds. Consider consuming these dense proteins less frequently and in small quantities.

In general—and there is no universal rule—the minimal amount of whole protein you require in a day can be calculated by dividing your ideal body weight by 15. That gives you the amount of protein required in ounces, which you would divide between your meals and snacks. For example, if your ideal body weight is 150 pounds, then you'd need a minimum of 10 ounces of whole protein over one day.

I am often asked if vegans and vegetarians get enough protein in their diets. I have to answer that question with a "maybe." Each of us is unique, and while some appear to do well on such diets, others do not. People who I have known to be very healthy on such diets devote a great deal of time and money toward the lifestyle and carefully calculate their nutritional intake every day. In general, I do not recommend diets devoid of any animal products, based on my clinical experience. I believe that the proteins and related nutrients obtained from foods such as eggs and fish, as well as meats such as buffalo and emu, can be very powerful for your health, even if eaten just a few times a week. You are unique. Learn and experiment, and you will find your balance.

Choosing the Right Carbs. Eating a variety of carbohydrates can provide a broad range of nutrients. Include vegetables, the most nutrient-rich carbohydrates, in every meal. Also consume a moderate amount of fruits, especially those with a low glycemic load (such as apples, pears, and peaches). Eat lightly cooked (preferably steamed) or raw vegetables to get the most out of their vitamin and mineral content. Vegetables lose their enzymes and nutrients when overcooked. Be careful with raw vegetables. They need to be washed thoroughly to get rid of harmful bacteria and parasites.

Eating a wide variety of carbohydrates also gives you a variety of fiber. Fiber, both soluble and insoluble, helps normalize bowel movements and digestion. Importantly, fiber slows the rate of entry of sugar into the bloodstream, thereby helping to maintain good blood sugar control. If you need extra fiber in your diet, add flaxseed meal and rice bran to your meals.

Most people associate "carbs" with bread, pasta, and other grain derived foods. These foods are highest in carbohydrate content per volume. As mentioned before, some of the healthiest people I have known ate no grains, but this does not mean you should jump on the bandwagon. If anything, reduce the amount of grain products you consume gradually and see how you feel. Some individuals may need more or less carbs and protein than others—and in the right balance—to feel mentally and physically renewed and energized. A skilled nutritionist can support you in determining the balance that is best for you.

When choosing the carbohydrate-rich foods that you want in your diet, consider the information in this chapter on glycemic control, as well as the gluten intolerance issue addressed in Chapter 6. Where grains are concerned, short-grain brown rice and millet are my personal favorites.

Choosing the Right Fats. Fat is probably the most maligned, misjudged, and misunderstood of all the macronutrients. The body needs quality sources of healthy fats—in sufficient amounts—to support many life-sustaining physiological functions.

Healthy fats are the building blocks for hormones and cell membranes, and are responsible for nerve conduction. Eaten in small quantities, they help control your weight by slowing down and regulating the rate at which sugar enters your bloodstream. This controlled release helps prevent blood sugar spikes that result in excess insulin secretion and fat storage.

Healthy fats take the form of monounsaturated fats, polyunsaturated fats, and saturated fats. Some good sources of monounsaturated fats include olive oil, hazelnuts, almonds, Brazil nuts, avocados, sesame seeds, and pumpkin seeds. Monounsaturated fats contain fatty acids that lower blood cholesterol by increasing the HDL (good) cholesterol and lowering the LDL (bad) cholesterol. Polyunsaturated fats are found in corn oil, flaxseed oil, hemp oil, safflower oil, sesame oil, and salmon oil, and in most cold water fish. They help to lower your total blood cholesterol by decreasing LDL cholesterol.

The two primary polyunsaturated fatty acids are omega-3 and omega-6. These fatty acids are known to contribute to reducing the risk of stroke, heart attack, and cancer. Omega-3 fatty acids are also known to reduce inflammation and lower triglyceride levels. Two essential fatty acids— alpha linolenic acid (ALA) and linolenic acid (LA)—are polyunsaturated oils that you need because your body cannot manufacture them. ALA is an omega-3 fatty acid and LA is an omega-6 fatty acid.

Maintaining a balance between omega-3 and omega-6 fatty acids in your diet is important, because both convert to chemicals involved in critical physiological processes. The recommended intake ratio for omega-6 to omega-3 is fraught with debate. While the most popular recommendation is 3:1, many health professionals are now advocating a ratio of 1:1. I advise maintaining this ratio between 1:1 and 3:1.

Omega-3 fatty acids include eicosapentaenoic acid (EPA) and docosahexanoic acid (DHA). Both are found primarily in oily cold water fish such as tuna, salmon, and mackerel. Aside from fresh seaweed, a staple of many cultures, plant foods rarely contain EPA or DHA.

Omega-3 fatty acids are also found in omega-3 eggs (from free-range chickens fed flaxseeds). Omega-6 fatty acids are found in avocados, eggs, sunflower oil, some nuts, seeds, and poultry. Almonds are another great source of omegas, and of protein, fiber, vitamin E, magnesium, and zinc. Beware that almonds are difficult for most people to digest because of an enzyme-inhibiting substance in their coating. Soaking the nuts for 12 hours removes this inhibitor to allow the enzymes secreted during digestion to do their job.

I recommend coconut oil for cooking, since it is not easily damaged by heat. Most oils, when heated to the point where they begin to smoke, lose their nutrient quality and oxidize, converting the original make-up of the oil to a substance not easily processed by the digestive system.

Saturated fats have been labeled "the bad guys," as they are incriminated as a contributing cause of heart disease. However, consuming a limited amount of high-quality saturated fat is actually beneficial. By my estimation, your daily caloric intake should be limited to less than 10 percent saturated fat. Saturated fat is found in meat and poultry, coconut oil, palm kernel oil, lard-pork fat, beef tallow, butter, and cocoa butter.

The following are a few important facts about saturated fats that

may surprise you:
- Saturated fats play a vital role in the health of our bones—at least 50 percent of our dietary fats need to be saturated for calcium to be incorporated effectively into the skeletal structure.
- Short- and medium-chain saturated fatty acids (found in ghee and coconut oil) have important antimicrobial properties, protecting us against harmful microorganisms in the digestive tract.
- They are needed for the proper utilization of essential fatty acids (EFAs).
- They constitute at least 50 percent of a cell's membrane, contributing to the cell's integrity.
- They protect the liver from the toxic effects of alcohol and certain drugs.

Trans fats (hydrogenated and partially hydrogenated), on the other hand, must be totally avoided. Oils like margarine and shortening are harmful because they turn into a trans fat during the process of hydrogenation. Trans fats are artificially altered to be solid at room temperature to preserve shelf life. Trans fats both raise bad (LDL) cholesterol and lower good (HDL) cholesterol. A high LDL cholesterol level in combination with a low HDL cholesterol level significantly increases the risk of heart disease, the leading cause of death for both men and women—a dietary double whammy that you must avoid.

pH—Health in the Balance

The measure of acidity or alkalinity of a solution is known as "pH," which stands for potential of hydrogen. The scale for measuring pH is from 0 to 14, with 7 being neutral. Below 7 is acidic; above 7 is alkaline. The optimal pH of the body's fluids, such as the blood and urine, is 7.4, slightly alkaline.

An acidic pH—referred to as acidosis—is caused by a diet of acid-forming foods, emotional stress, toxic overload, and any other process that deprives the cells of oxygen. The body will try to compensate for acidic pH by using alkaline minerals. If the diet does not contain enough minerals, a buildup of acids in the cells occurs, which impairs nutrient absorption and weakens the immune and detoxification systems. Acid buildup also impairs cellular energy production, promotes tumor cells, and increases the body's susceptibility to fatigue and illness. Furthermore, the depletion of minerals contributes to a long list of disorders, including arthritis, osteoporosis, and neurological impairment.

Acidosis is common in our society, given the typical diet that is far too high in acid-producing animal products like meat, eggs, and dairy, and far too low in alkaline-producing foods like fresh vegetables. Americans tend to eat acid-producing processed foods like white flour and sugar and drink acid-producing beverages like coffee and soft drinks. We also use too many prescription drugs and artificial sweeteners, both extremely acid-forming. One of the best things you can do to correct an overly acid body is to clean up your diet and lifestyle.

How Do I Stay Alkaline?

The process of pH balancing your body starts with diet and nutrition, including adequate hydration and eating a higher percentage of alkaline foods. As a general rule, your diet should consist of 60 percent alkaline-forming foods and 40 percent acid-forming foods. Alkaline-forming foods include most fruits, green vegetables, peas, beans, lentils, spices, herbs and seasonings, and seeds and nuts. Acid-forming foods include meat, fish, poultry, eggs, refined grains, sugar, some fruits (bananas and plums in particular), and processed foods.

Common foods that support an alkaline state include green vegetables, almonds, unpasteurized honey, bee pollen, maple syrup, figs, dates, goat and sheep dairy, root vegetables, apricots, avocados, coconut, grapes, molasses, raisins, and lemons.

Alkalinity is not just about what you eat but how you feel and think. Your emotions greatly influence the body's pH. Joyous, happy, love-filled emotions tend to create alkaline-forming chemical reactions in the body. Conversely, negative emotions such as anger, fear, jealousy, and hate create acid-forming chemical reactions in the body. This is done through the brain's master gland, the hypothalamus, which is controlled by our thoughts, emotions, and attitudes. This gland controls the entire hormonal system and the parasympathetic nervous system. With these systems out of synch, pH tends toward an acidic state.

One of the key factors is the water you drink. Unfortunately, most of the water we consume is acidic—including water treated with distillation, reverse osmosis, and deionization, all processes that remove minerals. Alkaline water is not readily available in most communities. However, you can solve this problem by adding minerals—in the form of unrefined sea salts—to your drinking water. Unrefined sea salt contains not only sodium chloride but also 80-plus trace elements and minerals from the ocean that are in perfect symbiosis with each other and the human body matrix. Unrefined sea salt offers a remarkable mineral balance relative to the internal environment of the human body. All of its elements are dosed naturally in proportions close to those of the internal human environment.

It is important to note that pH will not stabilize at an alkaline level on diet alone. If you are harboring chemicals or metals in your cells, you might tend toward an acidic state despite efforts to control pH through smart eating. This is also true if you have parasitic infections and inflammation.

Measuring pH

Being aware of the pH condition of your body is a good practice. You can measure your pH using urine or saliva. The test is simple and requires less than a minute of your time. Testing strips are available online and at your local drug store. Look for test strips that register half-point increments. When using these test strips as your guideline, balance the body pH between 7 and 7.5. If the test strips read above 7.5, consume acid-forming foods or beverages until it stabilizes between 7 and 7.5. While not always practical, the effort alone can greatly improve your health.

My Eight Simple Rules for Eating "Smart"

1. Eat five times a day. Eat a balanced breakfast, lunch, and dinner, and have two small snacks, one in the afternoon, and one around bedtime. Breakfast is the most important meal of the day; after all, you fasted all night. To maintain a balanced blood sugar level that provides energy throughout the day, make time to prepare a balanced meal in the morning. After four to five hours, you'll need another balanced meal or snack to replenish yourself and keep your blood sugar level steady. Some of us are better served by eating six or seven small meals throughout the day to maintain energy, prevent weight gain or muscle wasting, and stabilize blood sugar. Find what works for you with experimentation—and perhaps with the assistance of a skilled nutritionist.

2. Eat before you become hungry. Unfortunately, many people don't think about food until they're hungry. By that time, they're running out of fuel; that is, their blood sugar may already be low. Skipping meals also causes low blood sugar level.

3. Eat balanced meals and snacks. To recap, a balanced meal or snack consists of low-fat protein, low-glycemic carbohydrates, a smaller amount of high-glycemic "starchy" carbohydrates, healthy fats, and alkaline pH content. Avoid eating a large amount of carbohydrates without protein, as this will produce a sugar rush, then a crash. An hour or two later your blood sugar level will drop, and you will feel sluggish or irritable and experience difficulty thinking clearly.

4. Eat organic foods. One way to improve your nutritional status is to eat organic foods, which are richer in nutrients than commercially grown foods. Studies show that organically grown food contains a minimum of 50 to 100 percent more nutrients than commercially grown foods. Eating organic foods also eliminates the absorption of toxic pesticides, antibiotics, hormones, and herbicides found in commercially grown foods.

Be sure to wash produce thoroughly to rid them of dirt and undesirable organisms. I use the following procedure to clean produce:

1. Put ¼ to ½ cup of white, distilled vinegar into a large bowl of water.
2. Pre-wash the produce, place it into the bowl, and soak for 20 to 30 minutes.

3. Rinse a few times to remove the vinegar, then drain.

Store the produce in tightly sealed glass containers in the refrigerator; this will help maintain the food's freshness for up to four more days. Produce prepared in advance this way makes an excellent ready-to-eat, nutritious snack. As an extra food-handling precaution, equip your kitchen with separate cutting boards, one for meats and one for vegetables. This helps prevent contamination of produce with the harmful bacteria often found in raw meats. All cutting boards and knives that come into contact with meats should be thoroughly sanitized after every use.

5. Chew your food well. Take time to sit down and eat in a relaxed environment. Digestion begins with the sight, smell, and taste of food, and is enhanced as you chew. Primary digestion of carbohydrates begins in the mouth as enzymes in saliva mix with food. Our parents were right when they said, "Eat with your mouth closed and chew your food." This improves digestion and slows down the rate at which food converts to sugar and enters into the bloodstream.

Eating slowly, chewing thoroughly, and enjoying your meal in a calm setting improves digestion. The autonomic nervous system takes charge of digestion automatically. However, since it has two aspects that operate in a contrary manner—sympathetic and parasympathetic—the results of digestion can be either good or bad. When you are not focused on the act of eating—you are thinking about responsibilities at work or watching television, for example—the energy of digestion is diverted away from the activity of digestion. If you are emotionally charged while eating, then the sympathetic nervous system functioning dominates. The blood supply is sent to the peripheral muscles away from the stomach, digestive juices stop flowing, and the peristalsis of elimination stops. When the body and mind are at rest, the parasympathetic nervous system dominates and digestion and elimination proceed normally.

6. Avoid overeating. This is important. Would you overfill your gas tank? No, because doing so would waste gas and money. Overeating—filling your stomach beyond its capacity—creates indigestion, bloating, cramping, and that "stuffed" feeling. In reality, you are wasting food and money! If you are accustomed to overeating, practicing self-control is difficult in the beginning, but is well worth the effort in the end. Be certain to eat before you become hungry, as you will be less inclined to overeat.

7. Drink sufficient water. Drinking enough water is vital to maintaining your health. Water is the substance that bathes our cells and removes waste products. Unfortunately, most people don't drink enough water. When a person is chronically dehydrated, the thirst centers in the brain stop sending signals indicating their need for water. Most people who have been chronically dehydrated must consciously increase their intake of water for about one month to reestablish the normal firing of these thirst centers. Once you are rehydrated, normal thirst signals return.

The key to adequate hydration is to drink 100 percent water—no additives, no flavors, just water from the best sources. Beverages like coffee and soda dehydrate the body and deplete minerals. Fruit juice—with its accompanying spike in blood sugar levels—is certainly no substitute for water. Most people need a minimum of 64 ounces of water each day to ensure good digestive function, nerve conduction, and toxin elimination. Drinking a minimum of 8 to 16 ounces of water within 30 minutes of waking up is also a good idea, since you become slightly dehydrated during sleep.

As discussed in earlier chapters, I strongly recommend fresh, filtered water over plastic-bottled water. Look into home filtration and stainless steel containers for supplying yourself with less expensive, less wasteful, and more healthful drinking water.

8. Supplement with nutrient-dense formulas. Ideally, you would have flawless digestion, a steady metabolism, no oxidative stress, and strong detoxification capabilities. However, this is rarely the case. Even in our own kitchen, where my wife Joan and I maintain a fresh supply of organic produce and high-quality meats, nutritional supplements are in the cupboard and make up a daily regimen. Busy schedules, travel, and preexisting health factors prevent us from a well-rounded nutritional intake on a consistent basis (see www.biohealthinfo.com for resources).

On top of eating nutritious meals and snacks, I advise that you complement your diet with supplements containing therapeutic levels of bioavailable (easily absorbed) nutrients. B vitamins, vitamins C, D, and E, minerals, omega-rich oils, digestive enzymes, dense powders from fruits, herbs, vegetables, and more, can not only complete your daily nutrient intake, but make a positive difference in your body's ability to resist stress and remain in homeostasis. Just remember that they are called supplements for a reason; don't try to replace eating healthy, balanced meals with popping pills.

On a related note, if you are not already doing so, get a little exposure to natural sunlight daily. Too many people avoid it altogether for fear of developing skin cancer. Ten to fifteen minutes of exposure, in the morning or afternoon three to four times per week, is not only good for your adrenal glands, it boosts vitamin D. Such brief exposure will not increase your risk of skin cancer. If you lack adequate vitamin D, your body can absorb only a small amount of the calcium and only a little more than half of the phosphorus from your diet. Without adequate calcium and phosphorus, your bones will become brittle and break easily.

By following these simple rules and further educating yourself on food and nutrition, you can extend your life and increase your vitality. Remember: eating and drinking comes down to one choice at a time. Don't stress over it; simply learn what works for you and stay the course.

Sleeping to Recover

Ample rest for the body is critical, yet an estimated 68 percent of the United States population has insomnia. They take more than 20 minutes to fall asleep, they wake up periodically throughout the night, or they wake up and are unable to fall back to sleep. These sleep patterns fit the clinical definition of insomnia, a major source of chronic stress that promotes a Chronic Stress Response and compromises the hormone, immune, digestive, and detoxification systems.

Cortisol, DHEA, progesterone, melatonin, human growth hormone, estrogens, and testosterone all depend on quality sleep, as do neurotransmitters in the brain that can regenerate only with deep sleep. Poor sleep interferes with virtually all body functions and undermines homeostasis. You can't have optimal health and longevity if you are not sleeping well.

Disturbing the Internal Clock and Sleep Cycle. The hormone, immune, digestive, and detoxification systems are hardwired to your internal "clock," or circadian rhythm. The circadian clock in mammals is located in the hypothalamus. In modern society, we have chosen to ignore this basic law of nature, attempting to bend this physiological imperative to our own needs and desires. We pay a hefty price for doing so.

It's interesting to note that we live in a time where the days are extended with artificial light, which creates a shorter dark cycle. By shortening the dark cycle, we deprive ourselves of sleep. Try sleeping in a room that is completely dark. A dark sleeping environment supports the body's ability to regenerate. Another reason we are sleeping less, in addition to indoor lighting and multitasking lifestyles, is the universal acceptance and abuse of caffeine.

I am convinced that the multitude of caffeine junkies out there are caught in a vicious cycle of inadequate nightly recovery. The more caffeine you consume, the worse your sleep will be as a result of hormone disturbance, and your tendency to increase caffeine consumption rises, further robbing you of adequate sleep, and so on. If you insist on drinking coffee or other stimulants such as "energy" drinks, caffeinated teas, and sodas, limit your consumption to about 8 ounces and take these substances before noon, to minimize their interference with your sleep.

Poor blood sugar control may be a factor in your inability to rest and recover given the highs and lows at play with your nervous system and hormone levels. Exercise can support your ability to get a good night's sleep, or can interfere with it. Both overexercising—such as pushing yourself to run even when you're tired, injured, or experiencing pain—or exercising during times when you should be resting can feed this problem. Emotion is another lifestyle component that affects the quality of your sleep. If you are easily upset and carry around the negative emotions of the day, your mind will be busy and your body will be on alert. Learn to breathe deeply throughout the day and not internalize negative experiences.

Sleep and Immune Function. The immune system functions optimally if you are asleep by 10:00 P.M. Most physical repair takes place between approximately 10:00 P.M. and 2:00 A.M., when immune cells patrol your body, eliminating cancer cells, bacteria, viruses, and other harmful agents. Then, from about 2:00 to 6:00 A.M., you enter a stage of psychic or mental regeneration. During this time, the brain resets its chemical balance and releases substances that support the immune system. Throughout the night, you experience both rapid eye movement (REM) sleep states and non-REM stages, alternating between light sleep and deep dream states. This is how you process the mental and emotional events of the previous day and refresh your mind for the day ahead.

Most people need a minimum of seven to eight hours of sleep to accomplish all these tasks. Without sufficient sleep, the immune system is hard-pressed to keep up with its repair work, creating the opportunity for disease. Moreover, elevated cortisol at night from anxiety or the inability to fall asleep for other reasons may impair your immune functions.

Have you ever wondered why your cold or flu symptoms get worse at night? This happens because cortisol production regulates your immune system on a 24-hour cycle. As cortisol levels drop at night, your immune cells become highly active. The immune cells kill large numbers of bacteria and viruses, causing greater mucus production. As a result, you experience more congestion and coughing as your body attempts to get rid of the mucus. At daybreak, when cortisol levels rise, the activity of the immune cells tapers off. The immune cells then reset and recondition themselves to prepare for the next nightly cycle. This process is referred to as immune trafficking.

In addition to being the primary hormone that directs the immune function, cortisol dictates when we should be active and when we should rest. Cortisol levels follow a 24-hour cycle, peaking as the sun rises and tapering as the sun sets. As your cortisol levels rise, you're given the energy to begin your day. As they drop, reaching their lowest point about three hours after dark, your body enters a period of physical repair and psychic regeneration, which cannot happen with elevated cortisol levels. Staying awake beyond the time the body would naturally shut down keeps cortisol levels high, suppressing the release of human growth hormone and impeding the body's ability to repair and recover.

In 1910, the average adult slept nine to ten hours a night. Today, the average adult gets six to seven hours of this precious commodity. If you are in the latter camp, try getting to bed earlier, and limit the evening's barrage of lights, computers, and televisions, as this makes it that much harder for nature to take its course.

Exercise: Use It or Lose It

According to some surveys, less than 25 percent of the United States population exercises routinely. It's no wonder that we've become an unhealthy nation, considering the predominance of poor eating habits, lack of sleep, constant mental/emotional stress, and little or no exercise. One of the most effective ways to release tension, promote fat burning, improve immune function, and maintain balanced energy levels is by exercising.

This old saying is true about the body: "If you don't use it, you'll lose it." Your body was made to move, not to be sedentary. Movement is one of the keys to life and health. When you exercise, your breathing improves, bringing increased oxygen to your cells. Deep breathing and exercise move your lymph and cerebral spinal fluid, the fluidity of each being extremely important to immunity and nerve health. All of your body's fluids are designed to be in motion. Any and all exercise helps that process. The exercise doesn't have to be intense; one of the best forms of exercise is walking.

The following definition of exercise is from the American Medical Association Encyclopedia of Medicine: "The performance of any physical activity that improves health or that is used for recreation or correction of physical injury or deformity." Different types of exercise affect the body in one or more ways. Some improve flexibility, some improve muscular strength, some improve physical endurance, and some improve the efficiency of the cardiovascular and respiratory systems.

The Benefits of Routine Exercise

The topic of exercise, as well as the other topics in this chapter, could easily fill an entire book. Fortunately, there are plenty of exercise authors and trainers available to help you find a routine that works for you.

When to Work Out? Exercising first thing in the morning is optimal because you're rested and doing so will enhance your sense of energy and well-being for the rest of the day (assuming you don't overdo it). Have a light snack before your workout (e.g., almond butter and pear slices or water mixed with a powdered greens formula), since you are coming off hours of fasting. Sustaining an early morning exercise routine is often easier than an evening routine; you're tired at the end of the day and may have other things, like household chores and family activities, competing for your time.

What Types of Exercise? In general, exercise can be divided into three types of activities: cardiovascular such as running or bicycling; resistance training such as weightlifting; and flexibility, including stretching. Of course, many activities (soccer and swimming, for example), combine all three.

Cardiovascular exercise strengthens the heart and lungs and

contributes to improved circulation of blood and lymph throughout the body. Resistance exercise, besides strengthening muscle and building bone, can increase levels of human growth hormone (the hormone released by the pituitary gland that repairs and rebuilds body tissues) more than either cardiovascular or flexibility exercise. Since human growth hormone output declines with advancing age, it's especially important for individuals over 40 to include more resistance training. Flexibility exercises are noted for lowering stress hormone levels. All three types of activities should be included in your exercise routine to achieve the maximum health benefits, regardless of your age and health status. Incorporate and balance all three types regularly and safely.

Not Enough or Too Much? Exercise can just as easily be overdone as underdone. It's important to exercise appropriately to help relieve chronic stress, not add to it. Some symptoms of overexercising include joint pain, excessively sore muscles, stiffness, swelling, and decreased range of motion. Any of these symptoms is an indicator that your workout may have done more harm than good.

Regular, safe exercise increases the strength of muscles, bones, and connective tissues, allowing for enhanced mobility and independence as you age. Elderly people are especially inclined to become physically inactive and therefore lose joint mobility and bone mass, causing inflexibility and weakness. Rhythmic, gentle movement alone can help maintain a full range of movement of important joints, and even light exercises like walking can strengthen bones. Practices such as Qi Gong and yoga are tremendously beneficial to your whole being. By improving coordination and maintaining muscular strength, exercise reduces the risk of potential falls and related fractures commonly associated with aging.

As people become more sedentary, they also experience a decline in their cognitive function. Fortunately, at any age, there's usually some type of exercise that you can do. Even people who are wheelchair bound can often participate in water aerobics and other exercises. If you are able-bodied, yet have no valid excuses for not exercising... get moving!

Make It a Habit! I urge you to commit to a moderate cross-training exercise routine that is enjoyable and compatible with your interests. You will not only be healthier and improve the odds of living longer, but you will look more attractive and be mentally sharper. Exercise moderately—meaning don't be sedentary and don't overdo it. The extreme in either direction can feed the Chronic Stress Response.

Mental and Emotional Stress

While you can't always control what happens to you, you can control how you react to it. Channeling your emotions in a consciously positive way helps you to dramatically decrease the negative impact of stressful events. Learning how to do this is part of personal growth—mental and emotional, as well as spiritual. Integrating relaxation exercises such as meditation and deep breathing into your daily routine can make a dramatic improvement in your entire life, giving you the resolve to positively channel your emotions.

Mental and emotional responses to stimuli are referred to as limbic responses. The limbic system of the brain, sometimes called the "emotional nervous system," moderates your moods, maintains homeostasis, and helps form memories.

The Master Gland. The hypothalamus, a small gland at the base of the brain, is a principal limbic structure whose primary purpose is to maintain homeostasis in the body—meaning that it returns systems within your body to their "set points." Specifically, the hypothalamus regulates hunger, thirst, levels of pain and pleasure, sexual satisfaction, and aggressive or defensive behavior.

The hypothalamus—under the control of your thoughts, feelings, and attitudes—sends instructions through the autonomic nervous system and the pituitary gland. The autonomic nervous system regulates blood pressure, heart rate, breathing, digestion, and sweating, and serves other vital functions. The pituitary gland releases hormones that cause other endocrine glands, such as the adrenal glands and the thyroid, to secrete their hormones. The hypothalamus, therefore, is the principal intermediary between the nervous and endocrine systems—your body's two major control systems.

Fight or Flight. When under mental and emotional stress, the limbic system responds directly to the circumstances. Therefore, your perception and internalization of life's events can enhance or harm your health, based on the resulting limbic response. This is the essence of the mind/body connection.

Let's say you have a face-to-face encounter with a bear in the woods. Your brain immediately launches a fight-or-flight response, which stimulates your autonomic nervous system and triggers the response at the hormone level. Stress hormones like cortisol and adrenaline are released. When such a stress occurs repeatedly, this chronic overstimulation of your nervous system can lead to suppressed immunity and decreased energy because of the increased output of stress hormones. Recovering from a fight-or-flight response can be difficult, even traumatic.

Unfortunately, chronic overload of the autonomic nervous system is a common experience. Although you don't confront a bear every day, how many times have you hurried out the door in the morning to get to work on time? How often have you found yourself late for a meeting and stuck in rush-hour traffic or knee-deep in work that can't possibly be done on time? All of these events can create a fight-or-flight response that adversely affects your hormone, immune, digestive, and detoxification systems. Unfortunately, these types of stress can't be easily avoided in today's world. But you can control the way you respond to them.

Controlling Your Response to Stress. When you're under mental and emotional stress, a sequence of events occurs that determines how your body will respond physiologically:

1. First, you perceive the event.
2. Second, you respond to that event either positively or negatively.
3. Third, your thoughts and emotions internalize the event either positively or negatively.

This last step, internalization, is where problems can occur. If you respond negatively to an event, you'll likely internalize the experience negatively. Ultimately, this negative internalization—that is, holding on to the negative feelings generated by the stressful event—puts stressful demands on your nervous and endocrine systems.

Imagine that you're driving on the freeway and are suddenly forced onto the shoulder by a car that swerves into your lane. You barely miss being in a major accident. Typically, you have one of two responses:

- You may feel anger toward the driver who put your life in danger, internalizing the event and remaining upset for hours.
- You may feel relief that you avoided the accident and that no

one was injured. You may believe that the other driver either didn't see your car or was forced to turn to avoid another driver or an obstacle. Instead of negatively internalizing this event, you address it positively and carry on with your day.

It's clear which response might have a negative effect on your health. Remaining angry doesn't harm anyone except you—and perhaps those you unleash your negativity upon throughout the day. Internalizing the negative perception of an event is a major stress on the mind and body.

Multitasking. You can also stress your autonomic nervous system with excessive multitasking. This occurs when you change focus or shift attention too frequently, keeping your mind and body busy with multiple priorities and responsibilities.

For example, a young mother with two kids and a full-time job begins her day by getting the kids ready for school. The phone rings; it's the secretary from her office calling. The secretary informs her that a critical meeting set for 10 A.M. has been rescheduled for 9. Immediately after the mother hangs up the phone, one of the kids spills milk all over herself. The mother rushes to change her child's clothes and clean the mess, all the while mentally rearranging her day so she can run important errands after work instead of during the day and make it to her meeting on time. Most of these events are out of her control, and this level of multitasking and understandable frustration may cause her to feel mentally and emotionally overwhelmed. This young mother must address the problem or it will keep her in an ongoing fight-or-flight state.

Being able to think on your feet is great, but not to the point of collapse! The key is to find your balance point. If you're feeling mentally and emotionally overwhelmed, then you're not in balance. The answer? Reduce and control multitasking so you can restore balance to your autonomic nervous system.

The following are a few ways to minimize the stress created by multitasking:

- Keep a positive mental attitude and don't let challenges or failures get you down. Life's challenges don't feel so oppressive when you approach them calmly.
- Organize your schedule to allow yourself to focus on one thing at a time. Break up the day into reasonable chunks so you are doing one thing at a time. Get your most important tasks performed at the start of the day. Clear your physical and electronic in-boxes at the start of each day.
- Practice relaxation techniques such as diaphragmatic breathing, gentle stretching, yoga, t'ai chi, Qi Gong, meditation, biofeedback, and prayer. Make time for yourself. If you aren't true to your own needs, you can't help anyone else.
- Say "no" to people who may try to push you into a busier situation than you feel capable of handling efficiently. Explain that you have your limits, and preserve health and sanity first.
- Slow down. Much of the stress created by multitasking is from trying to go too fast. If you're rushing to get everything done, sit back, take a deep breath, and consider your true priorities. Write them down. Consider the routine tasks that you can delegate, eliminate, or outsource.
- Start your workday 15 to 30 minutes earlier, with a plan of spending that much more time at home or doing something you love.
- Write down your ideas on a portable notepad so they don't get lost in the mind's shuffle. Enter your ideas into a master

to-do list ranked in order of importance.

Life is filled with many challenges: mistakes that we make, mistakes other people make, accidents, people who don't agree with us, and people who don't want what we want. There are many things we can't control. By accepting this fact and relinquishing the desire to control every detail of your life and the lives of others, you can vastly reduce mental and emotional stress.

The Choices Are Yours

You have the power to improve your health and lengthen your life by making healthy lifestyle choices. Implementing small and consistent changes in how you live, think, and eat today can prevent illness and disease later. Time stops for no one. Prevention is the key. There are three things that must take place for you to experience positive lifestyle change.

- You must recognize the truth about your lifestyle habits. For example, "I'm not following good glycemic control and healthy diet choices."
- You must own this truth, accepting that it's your responsibility, as only you have the power to change your situation.
- You must take action. You can acknowledge truth and own it, but without taking action, nothing will change.

Don't delay. Start now! Make every day one filled with awareness and positive decisions. This is the most powerful thing you can do for your health and happiness. There are no magic pills or shots. There are no shortcuts. Doctors cannot help you if you don't help yourself. Evaluate how you can improve your lifestyle and take action—today, tomorrow, and for the rest of your life!

Epilogue

Get the Care You Deserve

Optimal health depends on smart lifestyle choices and receiving the best healthcare possible. Preventive care and an accurate diagnosis of any problem is the foundation. Inaccurate diagnoses inevitably lead to ineffective treatments. If treatment is symptom based, serious underlying problems may be masked, creating a dependency on symptomatic care and allowing life threatening dysfunctions to remain unaddressed. With an accurate diagnosis and a physician who knows how to interpret and apply this data, you can transcend the limits of symptomatic care.

A skilled doctor understands how the laboratory data from various tests "fit together" to form a comprehensive diagnostic analysis. Like the pieces of a puzzle, every bit of information is part of a broader picture. A thorough patient history and consideration of symptoms, together with laboratory findings, can guide a skilled clinician to the source of the problem.

Functional Diagnostic Medicine provides a roadmap for

discovering the root cause of health problems. It incorporates a logical sequence of functional lab assessments that examine the physiology of the body, specifically the interrelationships of the body's hormone, immune, digestive, and detoxification systems. These assessments can reveal the root causes of illness and disease.

A rapidly evolving specialty in medical diagnostics is radiology. In the last decade, breakthroughs in radiology have allowed doctors to literally look inside the body. Technologies like the CAT scan, MRI, and virtual colonoscopy have added a new dimension to medical diagnostic capabilities. Despite such advancements, these tools do not reveal the cause of disease. However, they are extremely useful at identifying a problem early in the disease process. This information, used in conjunction with functional diagnostic assessments, provides a powerful means to uncover the causes of potential—as well as existing—pathologies.

In this age of rapidly advancing technology, there is no justification for the needless suffering caused by an inadequate diagnosis and the treatment that results. Using affordable, state-of-the-art laboratory tests and therapies, optimal health outcomes are attainable. Whether fighting cancer, training for a sports competition, or seeking healthy longevity, an accurate assessment of your body's physiology can make all the difference.

Someone may have no symptoms and "suddenly" be diagnosed with a serious health condition. However, as you've seen, health problems rarely arise overnight. In fact, most are the result of imbalances in the body that have developed over years. Stress that becomes chronic in nature—that which results in a Chronic Stress Response—can develop into every illness and disease known to humans.

Years in the future, will we look back on today's practice of medicine as barbaric? Will the standard cancer treatments of today—poisoning with chemotherapy, surgically cutting out tumors, and burning with radiation—be perceived like the medieval practice of bloodletting?

It's up to each of us to take responsibility for our own health and embrace a healthy lifestyle. We also need to help reform our healthcare system by demanding from our elected officials the most effective and least harmful care. Stay abreast of the threats to health freedom by subscribing to alerts on state and federal legal actions that target human health. Most importantly—assuming you want to live long with vitality—breathe deeply, stand tall, and embrace each day with awareness and purpose. No one will do it for you, especially not doctors!

Purpose and Passion

Please take a moment to think about people you know who are happy and healthy. Do they have purpose and passion? If you lack purpose and passion, achieving optimal physical, mental, emotional, and spiritual health is difficult. What turns you on? What makes you happy? What makes you want to get out of bed and embrace the day? The importance of having purpose and passion in our lives cannot be overstated. A purposeful and passion-driven life is synonymous with optimal health.

I wrote this book to help you understand how your body reacts under stresses, both seen and hidden, and how your body's critical systems interrelate. I emphasize the importance of good lifestyle habits, and how they can prevent illness and improve health. I use functional lab assessments to discover the underlying cause of any health issue. Much of what I tell every single patient that seeks my help is said in this book for your benefit and for the benefit of the people you care about.

It's your life, your health, and your choice.

God bless and be well.

ONLINE RESOURCES

To locate health professionals utilizing Functional Diagnostic Medicine or to obtain general recommendations on the ideas, products, and services discussed in *The Chronic Stress Crisis,* please visit

www.biohealthinfo.com

References

Chapter Two: Diagnose and Treat the Cause, Not Just the Symptoms

Eriksen, B.O.; Kristiansen, I.S.; Nord, E.; Pape, J.F.; Almdahl, S.M.; Hensrud, A.; and Jaeger, S. The cost of inappropriate admissions: A study of health benefits and resource utilization in a department of internal medicine. *Journal of Internal Medicine*, October 1999; 246(4):379–87.

Hedley, A.A.; Ogden, C.L.; Johnson, C.L.; Carroll, M.D.; Curtin, L.R.; and Flegal, K.M. Overweight and obesity among US children, adolescents, and adults, 1999–2002. *Journal of the American Medical Association* 291:2847–2850.

Kohn, L.; Corrigan, J; and Donaldson, M., editors. *To Err Is Human: Building a Safer Health System*. Washington, DC: National Academy Press, 1999.

Schuster, M.; McGlynn, E.; and Brook, R. How good is the quality of healthcare in the United States? *Milbank Quarterly* 76 (1998):517–63.

Chapter Four: Adrenal Syndrome

Ferrari, E.; Cravello, L.; Muzzoni, B., et al. Age-related changes of the hypothalamic- pituitary-adrenal axis: Pathophysiological correlates. *European J Endocrinology*, April 2001; 144(4):319–29.

Janniere, L.; Canceill, D.; Suski, C.; Kanga, S.; Dalmais, B.; Lestini, R.; Monnier, A.F.; Chapuis, J.; Bolotin, A.; Titok, M.; Chatelier, E.L.; and Ehrlich, S.D. Genetic evidence for a link between glycolysis and DNA replication. *PLoS ONE*, May 16, 2007; 2:e447.

Lupien, S.; Lecours, A.R.; Lussoer, I.; Schwartz, G.; Nair, N.P.; and Meaney, M. Basal cortisol levels and cognitive deficits in human aging. *Journal of Neuroscience*, May 1994; 14(5 Pt 1):2893–903.

Chapter Five: The Mucosal Barrier: Your First-line Immune Defense

Magnusson, K.E., and Stjernström, I. Mucosal barrier mechanisms. Interplay between secretory IgA (SIgA), IgG and mucins on the surface properties and association of salmonellae with intestine and granulocytes. *Immunology*, February 1982; 45(2): 239–248.

Nash, T.E.; Herrington, D.A.; Losonsky, G.A.; and Levine, M.M. Experimental human infection with Giardia lamblia. *Journal of Infectious Diseases* 156 (1987): 974–84.

Rendtorff, R.C. The experimental transmission of human intestinal protozoan parasites. II *Giardia lamblia* cysts given in capsules. *American Journal of Hygiene* 59(1954): 209–20.

Veazey, R., and Lackner, A. The mucosal immune system and HIV-1 infection. *AIDS Rev.*, October–December 2003; 5(4):245–52.

Veazey R.S.; Marx, P.A.; and Lackner, A.A. The mucosal immune system: Primary target for HIV infection and AIDS. *Trends in Immunology*, November 2001; 22(11): 626–33.

Chapter Six: Bread: Staff of Life?

Bottaro, G.; Failla, P.; Rotolo, N.; Azzaro, F.; Spina, M.; Castiglione, N.; and Patane, R. The predictive value of antigliadin antibodies (AGA) in the diagnosis of non-celiac gastrointestinal disease in children. *Minerva Pediatr.*, March 1993; 45(3):93–98.

Cassidy, A., et al. Biological effects of a diet of soy protein rich in isoflavones on the menstrual cycle of premenopausal women. *American Journal of Clinical Nutrition* 60 (1994):333–40.
52.

Counts, D.R., and Sierpina, V.S. Celiac disease/ gluten intolerance. *Explore*, July–August 2006; 2(4):291.

Guarner, F., and Malagelada, J. Gut flora in health and disease. *The Lancet* 361, Issue 9356, 512–19.

Hourigan, C.S. The molecular basis of coeliac disease. *Clin Exp Med*, June 2006; 6(2):53–59.

Kagnoff, M.F. Mucosal inflammation in celiac disease: Interleukin-15 meets transforming growth factor beta-1. *Gastroenterology*, March 2007; 132(3):1174–76.

Lahdeaho, M.L.; Kaukinen, K.; Collin, P.; Ruuska, T.; Partanen, J.; Haapala, A.M.; and Maki, M. Celiac disease: From inflammation to atrophy: a long-term follow-up study. *Journal of Pediatric Gastroenterol Nutr*, July 2005; 41(1):44–48.

Loginov, A.S.; Parfenov, A.I.; Vasil'ev, A.V.; Chikunova, B.Z.; and Parfenov, D.A. The potentials of intestinoscopy and guided biopsy in the diagnosis of diseases of the small intestine. *Ter Arkh*, 1999; 71(2):31–37.

Murphy, P.A. Phytoestrogen content of processed soybean foods. *Food Technology*, January 1982, 60–64.

Chapter Seven: Your Body's Uninvited Guests

Dagci, H., et al. Protozoan infections and intestinal permeability. *Acta Trop*, January 2002; 81(1):1–5.

Ertug, S., et al. The effect of blastocystis hominis on the growth status of children. *Medical Science Monitor*, December 18, 2006; 13(1):CR40–43.

Follett, R.H., and Self, J.R. Domestic water quality criteria. Colorado State University Cooperative Extension, Service in Action, 513, Fort Collins, CO, 1989.

Fundingsland, S., and Lundstrom, D. Drinking Water and Health. Pub. 27, HEA, NDSU Extension Service, North Dakota State University, Fargo, ND 58105, June 1988.

Green, L.R.; Radke, V.; Mason, R.; Bushnell, L.; Reimann, D.W.; Mack, J.C.; Motsinger, M.D.; Stigger, T.; and Selman, C.A. Factors related to food worker hand hygiene practices. *Journal of Food Protection*, March 2007; 70(3):661–66.

Guerrant, R.L. Cryptosporidiosis: an emerging, highly infectious threat. *Emerg Infect Dis.*, January–March 1997; 3(1):51–57.

Hunter, P.R.; Hadfield, S.J.; Wilkinson, D.; Lake, I.R.; Harrison, F.C.; and Chalmers, R.M. Subtypes of Cryptosporidium parvum in humans and disease risk. *Emerg Infect Dis.*, January 2007; 13(1):82–88.

Konturek P.C.; Konturek, S.J.; and Brzozowski, T. Gastric cancer and Helicobacter pylori infection. *Journal of Physiological Pharmacology*, September 2006; 57 Suppl. 3:51–65.

Li, E., and Stanley, S.L. Jr. Protozoa. Amebiasis. *Gastroenterol Clin of North America*, September 1996; 25(3):471–92.

Norberg, A.; Nord, C.E.; and Evengard, B. Dientamoeba fragilis— a protozoal infection which may cause severe bowel distress. *Clinical Microbiol Infect*, January 2003; 9(1):65–68.

Frank Nova, MD, Chief of the Laboratory for Parasitic Diseases of the National Institute of Health: "In terms of numbers there are more parasitic infections acquired in this country than in Africa."

Pajares, J.M., and Gisbert, J.P. Helicobacter pylori: Its discovery and relevance for medicine. *Rev Esp Enferm Dig*, October 2006; 98(10):770–85.

Stanley, S.L. Jr. Amoebiasis. *Lancet*, March 22, 2003; 361(9362):1025–34.

Stark, van Hal, Marriott, Ellis, and Harkness. Irritable bowel syndrome: A review on the role of intestinal protozoa and the importance of their detection and diagnosis. *International Journal for Parasitology* 37 (2007), 11–20.

Walsh, J.A. *Rev. Infect. Dis.* 8 (1988), 228–38.

Yakoob, J.; Jafri, W.; et al. Irritable bowel syndrome: In search of an etiology: role of Blastocystis hominis. *American Journal of Trop. Med. Hyg.* 70(4), 2004, 383–85.

Chapter Eight: The Mold Effect

Berek, L.; Petri, I.B.; Mesterhazy, A.; et al. Effects of mycotoxins on human immune functions in vitro. *Toxicology In Vitro* 15 (2001):25–30

Gray, M. Molds and mycotoxins: Beyond allergies and asthma.

Alternative Ther Health Med, March–April 2007; 13(2):S146–52.

Kilburn, K.H. Inhalation of moulds and mycotoxins. *European Journal of Oncology*, 7 (2002):197–202.

Lee, T.G. Health symptoms caused by molds in a courthouse. *Arch Environmental Health*, July 2003; 58(7):442–46.

Savilahti, R.; Uitti, J.; Laippala, P.; et al. Respiratory morbidity among children following renovation of water-damaged school. *Arch Environmental Health* 55 (2000):405–10.

Vesper, S.J.; McKinstry, C.; Yang, C.; Haugland, R.A.; Kercsmar, C.M.; Yike, I.; Schluchter, M.D.; Kirchner, H.L.; Sobolewski, J.; Allan, T.M.; and Dearborn, D.G. Specific molds associated with asthma in water-damaged homes. *Journal of Occupational Environmental Medicine*, August 2006; 48(8):852–58.

Wall Street Journal, page 1, January 9, 2007. "Amid Mold Suits, Experts Wear Two Hats."

Chapter Nine: Heavy Metal Toxicity

Agency for Toxic Substances and Disease Registry (ATSDR). Annual Report, July 1999.

Baskin, D.S.; Ngo, H.; and Didenko, V.V. Thimerosal indices, DNA breaks, caspase-3 activation, membrane damage, and cell death in cultured human neurons and fibroblast. *Toxicology Science* 74 (2003): 361–68.

Blaylock, R. Interaction of cytokines, excitotoxins, and reactive nitrogen and oxygen species in autism spectrum disorders. *Journal of the American Nutrition Association* 6 (2003): 21–35.

Drasch, G.; Schupp, I.; Hofl, H.; Reinke, R.; and Roider, G. Mercury burden of human fetal and infant tissues. *European Journal of*

Pediatrics 153 (1994): 607–10.

Foster, H.D. How aluminum causes Alzheimer's disease. *Journal of Orthopedic Medicine* 15 (1) (2000): 21–51.

Geier, D.A., and Geier, M.R. A comparative evaluation of the effects of MMR immunization and mercury doses from thimerosalcontaining childhood vaccines on the population prevalence of autism. *Medical Science Monitor*. March 2004; 10(3):PI33-9. Epub March 1, 2004.

Hilliard-Lysen, J., and Riemer, J.W. Occupational stress and suicide among dentists. *Deviant Behavior* 9 (1988):333–46.

Koos et al., Mercury toxicity in pregnant women, fetus and newborn infants. American *Journal of Obstetrics and Gynecology*, 126 (1976):390–409.

McLachlan, D.R., et al. Brain desferroxamine in patients with Alzheimer's disease. *Lancet*, 337 (1991): 1304–8.

Morgan, R.E.; Garavan, H.; et al. Early lead exposure produces lasting changes in sustained attention, response initiation, and reactivity to errors. *Neurotoxicology and Teratology* 23 (2001): 519–31.

Stack, S. Suicide risk among dentists: A multivariate analysis. *Deviant Behavior* 17 (1996):107–18.

Tezel, H., et al. Blood mercury levels of dental students and dentists at a dental school. *British Dentistry Journal* 191 (2001): 449–52.

Chapter Ten: Chemically Stressed?

American Thoracic Society. Children living near major roads at higher asthma risk. *Science Daily*, 2004.

Dominici, F.; Peng, R.D.; Bell, M.L.; Pham, L.; McDermott, A.;

Zeger, S.L.; and Samet, J.M. Fine particulate air pollution and hospital admission for cardiovascular and respiratory diseases. *Journal of the American Medical Association*, March 8, 2006 (10):1127–34.

Glinton, G.J. Multiple-chemical sensitivity. *Medsurg Nursing*, December 2005 (6):365–69.

Hansen, O.G. PVC and phthalates in medical devices: A never ending story. *Medical Device Technology*, April 2006; 17(3):16–18.

Ishibashi, M.; Tonori, H.; Miki, T.; Miyajima, E.; Kudo, Y.; Tsunoda, M.; Sakabe, K.; and Aizawa, Y. Classification of patients complaining of sick house syndrome and/or multiple chemical sensitivity. *Tohoku Journal of Experimental Medicine*, March 2007; 211(3):223–33.

Journal of Applied Nutrition. Organic food is more nutritious than conventional food; 45 (1993):35–39.

Kleinsasser, N.H.; Kastenbauer, E.R.; Wallner, B.C.; Weissacher, H.; and Harreus, U.A. Genotoxicity of phthalates. On the discussion of plasticizers in children's toys. *HNO*, May 2001; 49(5):378–81.

Latini, G.; De Felice, C.; and Verrotti, A. Plasticizers, infant nutrition and reproductive health. *Reproductive Toxicology*, November 2004; 19(1):27–33.

National Cancer Policy Board. "Making Better Drugs for Children with Cancer" (2005).

Pelley, J. Acid rain worries in western Canada. *Environmental Science Technology*, October 1, 2006; 40(19):5830.

Sorahan, T.; Burges, D.C.; Hamilton, L.; and Harrington, J.M. Lung cancer mortality in nickel/chromium platers, 1946–95. *Occupational Environmental Medicine*, April 1998; 55(4):236–42.

Tschirley, F.H. Dioxin. *Scientific American* 254 (February 1986), 34.

Chapter Eleven: Electromagnetic Radiation

Cech, R.; Leitgeb, N.; and Pediaditis, M. Fetal exposure to low frequency electric and magnetic fields. *Phys Med Biol*, February 21, 2007; 52(4):879–88. Epub, January 17, 2007.

Fernandez-Sola, J.; Lluis Padierna, M.; Nogue Xarau, S.; and Munne Mas, P. Chronic fatigue syndrome and multiple chemical hypersensitivity after insecticide exposure. *Med Clin (Barc)*, April 2, 2005; 124(12):451–53.

Goodman and Blank. Magnetic field stress induces expression of hsp70. *Cell Stress & Chaperones*, 1998, 3(2), 79–88.

Malkin, R.A., and Hoffmeister, B.K. AC leakage currents cause complete hemodynamic collapse below the ventricular fibrillation threshold. *Computers in Cardiology*, 1999:351–53.

Mirick, D.K.; Chen, C.; and Stevens, R.G. Residential magnetic fields, light-at-night, and nocturnal urinary 6-sulfatoxymelatonin concentration in women. *American Journal of Epidemiology*, October 1, 2001; 154(7):591–600.

NTP Toxicology and Carcinogenesis Studies of 60-HZ Magnetic Fields IN F344/N Rats and B6C3F1 Mice (Whole-body Exposure Studies). *National Toxicology Program Tech Rep Ser*, April 1999; 488:1–168.

Pira, E.; Zanetti, C.; and Saia, B. Carcinogenic risk of extremelylow-frequency electromagnetic fields: State of the art. *Med Lav*, November–December 1994; 85(6):447–62.

Repacholi, M.H.; Basten, A.; Gebski, V.; Noonan, D.; Finnie, J.; and Harris, A.W. Lymphomas in E mu-Pim1 transgenic mice exposed to pulsed 900 MHZ electromagnetic fields. *Radiat Res*, May 1997; 147(5):631–40.

Repacholi, M.H. Low-level exposure to radiofrequency

electromagnetic fields: Health effects and research needs. *Bioelectromagnetics*, 1998, 19(1):1–19.

Stoupel, E.; Domarkiene, S.; Radishauskas, R.; and Abramson, E. Sudden cardiac death and geomagnetic activity: Links to age, gender and agony time. *Journal of Basic Clinical Physiological Pharmacology*, 2002; 13(1):11–21.

Vignati, M., and Giuliani, L. Radiofrequency exposure near highvoltage lines. *Environmental Health Perspectives*, December 1997; 105 Suppl 6:1569–73.

Chapter Twelve: Trauma, Inflammation, and Pain

Guyton, Hall. *Textbook of Medical Physiology*, 2001.

Helm, et al. Stress, childhood trauma linked to chronic fatigue syndrome in adults. *Arch Gen Psychiatry*, 2006; 63:1258–66 and 1267–72.

Inoue, M.; Kitakoji, H.; Ishizaki, N.; Tawa, M.; Yano, T.; Katsumi, Y.; and Kawakita, K. Relief of low back pain immediately after acupuncture treatment—a randomized, placebo controlled trial. *Acupuncture Medicine*, September 2006; 24(3):103–8.

Lude, P.; Kennedy, P.; Evans, M.; Lude, Y.; and Beedie, A. Post traumatic distress symptoms following spinal cord injury: A comparative review of European samples. *Spinal Cord*, February 2005; 43(2):102–8.

Part III: The Four Lifestyle Factors

Asami, D., et al. Comparison of the total phenolic and ascorbic content of freeze-dried and air-dried marionberry, strawberry, and corn grown using conventional, organic, and sustainable agricultural practices. *Journal of Agricultural and Food Chemistry*, 2003;

51(5):1237–41.

Bonnet, M.H., and Arand, D.L. Situational insomnia: Consistency, predictors, and outcomes. *Sleep*, December 15, 2003; 26(8):1029–36.

Buchner, D.M.; Beresford, S.A.A.; Larson, E.B.; LaCroix, A.; and Wagner, E.H. Effects of physical activity on health status in older adults II: Intervention studies. *Annual Review of Public Health* 13 (1992), 469–88.

Carlson, L.E.; Speca, M.; Patel, K.D.; and Goodey, E. Mindfulness-based stress reduction in relation to quality of life, mood, symptoms of stress and levels of cortisol, dehydroepiandrosterone sulfate (DHEA-S) and melatonin in breast and prostate cancer outpatients. *Psychoneuroendocrinology*, May 2004; 29(4):448–74.

CDC National Center for Chronic Disease. Number of Americans with diabetes continues to increase. October 26, 2005.

Gais, S.; Lucas, B.; and Born, J. Sleep after learning aids memory recall. *Learning and Memory*, May–June 2006; 13(3):259–62.

Harvard University. Carbohydrates and health: Not that simple ...or that complex. Taking control of your blood sugar and insulin levels may pay off for your heart and overall health. *Harvard Heart Letter*, December 2002; 13(4):3–4.

Lau, C.; Faerch, K.; Glumer, C.; Tetens, I.; Pedersen, O.; Carstensen, B.; Jorgensen, T.; and Borch-Johnsen, K. Dietary glycemic index, glycemic load, fiber, simple sugars, and insulin resistance. *Diabetes Care*, June 2005; 28(6):1397–403.

Lewis, S. Broken heart syndrome: Perspectives from East and West. *Adv Mind Body Med*, Summer 2005; 21(2):3–5.

Mayo Clinic. Amount of sleep linked to coronary artery disease risk. *Mayo Clinic Women's Healthsource*, July 2003; 7(7):3.

Mokdad, A.H., et al. Actual causes of death in the United States, 2000. *Journal of the American Medical Association* 291(10): 1238–45.

Monnikes, H., et al. Role of stress in functional gastrointestinal disorders. Evidence for stress-induced alterations in gastrointestinal motility and sensitivity. *Digestive Disorders*, 2001; 19(3):201–11.

Pedersen, B.K., and Hoffman-Goetz, L. Exercise and the immune system: Regulation, integration, and adaptation. *Physiology Review*, July 2000; 80(3):1055–81.

Roth, T. Prevalence, associated risks, and treatment patterns of insomnia. *Journal of Clinical Psychiatry*, 2005; 66 Suppl 9:10-3.

Rozanski, A.; Blumenthal, J.A.; and Kaplan, J. Impact of psychological factors on the pathogenesis of cardiovascular disease and implications for therapy. *Circulation*, April 27, 1999; 99(16):2192–217.

Sahyoun, N.R.; Anderson, A.L.; Kanaya, A.M.; Koh-Banerjee, P.; Kritchevsky, S.B.; de Rekeneire, N.; Tylavsky, F.A.; Schwartz, A.V.; Lee, J.S.; and Harris, T.B. Dietary glycemic index and load, measures of glucose metabolism, and body fat distribution in older adults. *American Journal of Clinical Nutrition*, September 2005; 82(3):547–52.

Sleep Disorders Institute. Annual Report of the Trans-NIH Sleep Research Coordinating Committee, 2002.

Srinivasan, V.; Maestroni, G.; et al. Melatonin, immune function and aging. *Immunology of Ageing*, November 2005; 2:17.

Surgeon General. Physical Activity and Health. National Center for Chronic Disease Prevention and Health Promotion, 1999.

Wagner, E.H., and Lacroix, A.Z. Effects of physical activity on health status in older adults I: Observational studies. *Annual Review of Public Health* 13 (1992), 451–68.

Worthington, V. Nutritional quality of organic versus conventional fruits, vegetables, and grains. *The Journal of Alternative and Complementary Medicine*, 2001; 7(2) 161–73.

D.K.; Miller, N.H.; and Debusk, R.F. Effects of low- and highintensity home-based exercise training on functional capacity in healthy middle-age men. *American Journal of Cardiology* 57 (1986), 446–49.

Index

A

ACTH 64
Addison's disease 48, 59
Adrenal exhaustion 48, 55, 59, 60, 61, 62, 83
Adrenal glands xiv, 29, 46, 47, 52, 56, 59, 60, 62, 64, 65, 66, 67, 164, 191, 199
Adrenal syndrome 59, 60, 62, 63, 67, 163, 164, 166, 212
Air filter 114
Air pollution 9, 45, 138, 218
Aldosterone 29, 47, 50
Allergies 2, 4, 6, 19, 26, 45, 60, 61, 62, 71, 84, 95, 122, 138, 215
Alpha linolenic acid 182
Aluminum 9, 11, 119, 128, 129, 130, 217
Aluminum exposure, sources 129
Amalgam fillings 7, 14, 51, 126
Antigen overload 72
Antigens 71, 72, 75, 84
Antioxidants 119, 145
Anxiety 4, 43, 44, 45, 50, 55, 60, 61, 63, 169, 176, 179, 194
Arsenic 119, 127, 128
Arsenic exposure, sources 127, 128
Asthma 138, 215, 216, 217
Auto-immune disease 45, 72, 73, 75, 80, 93, 94, 98, 165

B

Bacteria 29, 53, 71, 72, 85, 86, 93, 97, 98, 101, 103, 108, 121, 181, 189, 194
Benzene 135, 140
Biofeedback 3, 166, 167, 170, 202
Blastocystis hominis 73, 92, 101, 102, 214, 215
Bob Timmins 3, 167
Bone 30, 48, 119, 124, 126, 129, 165, 176, 197
Brain 13, 14, 20, 29, 48, 52, 63, 64, 65, 85, 86, 96, 104, 105, 115, 124, 129, 136, 143, 152, 164, 170, 173, 176, 179, 186, 190, 192, 194, 198, 199, 217

C

Cadmium 119, 125, 126
Cadmium exposure, sources 126
Cancer xiv, xv, 23, 26, 31, 33, 38, 39, 45, 53, 86, 87, 88, 95, 100, 122, 127, 128, 137, 141, 151, 152, 153, 154, 155, 157, 165, 176, 182, 191, 193, 206, 207, 214, 218, 221
Candida 55, 86, 93
Carbohydrates 23, 31, 50, 66, 86, 175, 176, 177, 178, 179, 180, 181, 188, 189, 221
Carbon filters 142
Cardiovascular disease 33, 45, 176, 222
Cell mediated immunity 30
Chelation 131, 146
Chemical exposure, sources 19, 133, 134, 139
Chemical hypersensitivity 12, 16, 219
Chemicals 4, 5, 7, 10, 11, 12, 14, 15, 17, 30, 45, 51, 53, 65, 98, 107, 112, 118, 131, 133, 134, 135, 136, 137, 138, 139, 140, 141, 143, 144, 145, 146, 147, 153, 182, 187
Chemotherapy 38, 207
Chronic fatigue 24, 33, 54, 55, 82, 83, 93, 113, 122, 135, 155, 169, 219, 220
Chronic stress xiii, xiv, 13, 14, 17, 19, 20, 25, 26, 32, 34, 43, 44, 47,

225

50, 51, 53, 56, 60, 61, 64, 70, 71, 75, 79, 80, 84, 91, 96, 102, 103, 109, 111, 118, 130, 134, 153, 155, 158, 159, 164, 165, 169, 170, 192, 197
Chronic stress response xix, 13, 14, 18, 19, 20, 21, 28, 31, 37, 43, 44, 47, 49, 51, 53, 57, 60, 63, 73, 80, 103, 104, 110, 130, 132, 133, 143, 147, 151, 159, 163, 166, 174, 192, 198, 206
Circadian rhythm 66, 192
Clostridium difficile 92, 103
Cortisol 13, 29, 47, 48, 49, 50, 51, 52, 53, 60, 63, 64, 65, 66, 67, 71, 91, 163, 164, 176, 192, 194, 195, 199, 212, 221
Cortisol to DHEA ratio 63, 64, 65, 192
Cortisone 29, 52
Cow's milk dairy 88
Crohn's disease 72, 122, 123
Cryptosporidium parvum 55, 73, 92, 99, 214

D

Dental fillings 14, 120
Depression 33, 45, 49, 54, 55, 60, 61, 62, 63, 82, 83, 93, 98, 121, 124, 135, 138, 155, 169, 173
Detoxification 11, 13, 14, 15, 16, 28, 31, 32, 39, 48, 53, 55, 56, 66, 72, 82, 96, 130, 131, 146, 158, 185, 191, 192, 200, 206
DHEA 29, 47, 48, 49, 51, 60, 63, 64, 65, 66, 67, 71, 192, 221
Diarrhea 10, 74, 80, 92, 97, 98, 99, 103, 113, 122, 124
Dientamoeba fragilis 92, 103, 215
Diet xiii, xiv, 4, 7, 8, 16, 23, 33, 34, 37, 45, 83, 84, 85, 87, 88, 89, 93, 145, 173, 174, 175, 181, 182, 185, 187, 191, 203, 213
Diets 86, 88, 89, 175, 180
Digestive function 190

Digestive system 126, 183
Dioxin 136, 137, 218

E

Eating 8, 39, 79, 81, 86, 89, 94, 137, 139, 140, 173, 175, 176, 178, 179, 180, 181, 185, 187, 188, 189, 191, 192, 195
Electromagnetic radiation 149, 150, 151, 152, 156, 159, 219
Emotional and mental trauma 45, 46, 51, 174, 195, 198, 199, 200, 203
Endocrine system 59
Entamoeba histolytica 73, 92, 95, 96
Environmental illness xvii, 5, 6, 7, 11, 12, 16, 133
Essential fatty acids 182, 184
Estradiol 29, 49
Estriol 29, 49
Estrogens 29, 47, 49, 192
Estrone 29, 49
Exercise xiii, 16, 19, 32, 33, 34, 37, 44, 45, 46, 50, 144, 166, 173, 174, 193, 195, 196, 197, 198, 222, 223

F

Fast food 140
Fatigue 21, 24, 32, 33, 44, 46, 51, 54, 55, 61, 62, 63, 67, 80, 82, 83, 93, 103, 105, 109, 113, 115, 122, 124, 135, 155, 169, 173, 176, 179, 185, 219, 220
Fats 23, 31, 85, 86, 97, 98, 144, 175, 179, 181, 182, 183, 184, 188
First-line immunity 70, 74, 106
Food allergies 19, 60, 61, 84, 122
Food intolerances 31, 44
Food proteins 71
Foods to avoid on a gluten free diet 83, 88, 89
Free radicals 144, 145
Functional diagnostic 82, 206

Functional Diagnostic ix, xviii, 20, 26, 37, 41, 67, 205, 209
Functional diagnostic testing 82, 206
Fungi 71, 85, 86, 111, 115, 121

G

Gastrointestinal system 87, 106
Gauss meter 155, 158
Geophysical stress 45
Giardia lamblia 55, 73, 74, 92, 97, 212
Gliadin 16, 73, 79, 80, 87, 89
Glucagon 175, 177
Gluconeogenesis 52
Glucose 51, 52, 65, 66, 175, 176, 222
Gluten-free 83, 87, 88, 89
Gluten intolerance 45, 50, 55, 73, 79, 80, 81, 83, 84, 85, 86, 89, 90, 97, 165, 181, 213
Glycemic control 51, 52, 181, 203
Glycemic index 176, 177, 178, 179, 221, 222
Glycemic load 176, 177, 178, 179, 181, 221

H

Hair loss 61, 124, 128
HCL, hydrochloric acid 23, 73, 100
Heart v, 20, 21, 22, 27, 28, 32, 39, 40, 41, 52, 61, 85, 105, 124, 138, 151, 164, 182, 183, 184, 196, 199, 221
Heavy Metals 16, 24, 39, 130, 131, 132, 146
Heavy metal toxicity 24, 119, 130, 131, 132, 146, 216
Heavy metal toxicity, diagnosing 131
Helicobacter pylori 23, 40, 46, 92, 100, 101, 108, 214, 215
High blood sugar 176
HIV 53, 72, 74, 99, 212, 213
Homeostasis 25, 26, 28, 44, 176, 191, 192, 198, 199
Homeostasis, and five stages of disorder 26
Hormone imbalance 46, 47, 83
Hormones xiv, 19, 28, 29, 47, 48, 49, 59, 60, 63, 66, 67, 71, 83, 134, 140, 175, 182, 188, 199
Human growth hormone 54, 56, 66, 192, 195, 197
Humoral immunity 30
Hypermotility 55, 85, 97
Hypothalamus 29, 64, 186, 192, 198, 199

I

Immune cells 52, 53, 65, 165, 193, 194
Immune complex 72
Immune trafficking 194
Immunity 23, 30, 52, 55, 59, 65, 70, 72, 74, 75, 98, 99, 106, 122, 195, 199
Immunocytes 65, 71
Immunoglobulins 52, 65, 71
Infectious agents 30, 53, 65, 70, 72, 94, 164
Inflammation 31, 40, 45, 53, 62, 70, 72, 73, 80, 85, 86, 97, 99, 105, 110, 163, 164, 165, 166, 168, 170, 182, 187, 213, 220
Inflammatory bowel disease 72, 96, 122
Injury 19, 128, 163, 164, 169, 196, 220
Insomnia 33, 44, 50, 60, 82, 123, 155, 169, 192, 221, 222
Insulin 29, 51, 175, 176, 177, 182, 221
Irritability 62, 109, 122, 124
Irritable Bowel Syndrome 102, 215

L

Lab testing xiii, 28, 29, 33, 34, 46, 53, 98, 130
Lacteals 85
Lactose 45, 84, 87, 97

Lactose intolerance 45
Lead 19, 38, 45, 48, 51, 65, 119, 124, 125, 164, 165, 199, 205, 217
Lead exposure, sources 124, 125, 217
Light cycle disruption 45
Linolenic acid 182
Liver xviii, 32, 52, 55, 62, 65, 66, 72, 95, 96, 97, 98, 123, 124, 126, 127, 128, 141, 168, 184
Low blood sugar 60, 176, 188
Lymphocytes 30, 53, 112

M

Malabsorption 45, 55, 80, 85, 99
Malnutrition 55, 85, 157
Medical intervention 21, 22, 24, 27, 37, 41, 54, 56, 82
Menopause 83, 87
Menstrual difficulties 50
Mercury 7, 14, 38, 51, 119, 120, 121, 122, 216, 217
Mercury exposure, sources 121
Metabolism 47, 48, 59, 66, 115, 126, 176, 191, 222
Methylmercury from fish consumption 121
Microvilli 84, 85
Mold 45, 111, 112, 113, 114, 115, 116, 117, 118, 215, 216
Mold contamination 112
Mold problems in public buildings 118
Molds 7, 111, 112, 113, 114, 115, 116, 117, 118, 215, 216
Mood swings 62, 121
Mucosal antibodies 71
Mucosal barrier 30, 31, 52, 53, 69, 70, 71, 72, 73, 74, 75, 80, 85, 94, 97, 98, 99, 106, 123, 212
Mucosal Immunity 30, 75, 98
Mucous plugs 85, 87, 97
Multitasking xiii, 193, 201, 202
Muscle xiii, 10, 48, 49, 52, 61, 65, 80, 82, 93, 96, 105, 122, 124, 129, 157, 165, 167, 176, 188, 197

Mycotoxins 115, 215, 216

N

Natural killer (NK) cells 30, 53
Nervous system 25, 52, 64, 94, 98, 124, 127, 129, 136, 141, 186, 189, 190, 193, 198, 199, 201, 202
Neurological 15, 98, 113, 121, 127, 185
Neurotoxins 98, 112
Nickel 38, 119, 122, 123, 126, 218
Nickel, exposures 122, 123
Nickel toxicity 122
Nutritional products 39

O

Organic 11, 82, 107, 111, 112, 115, 116, 128, 139, 140, 188, 191, 218, 220, 223
Osteoporosis 82, 83, 86, 119, 185
Ovaries 29, 67
Oxidative stress 119, 144, 145, 191

P

Pain xv, 3, 10, 14, 21, 22, 23, 24, 32, 34, 35, 45, 61, 62, 80, 86, 103, 105, 120, 122, 124, 126, 146, 163, 164, 165, 166, 167, 168, 170, 193, 197, 199, 220
Pain, acute 35, 164
Pain, chronic 3, 86, 166, 167
Parasite – definition 91
Pathogen – definition 93
Pathogens 30, 52, 53, 65, 71, 87, 103
Pesticides 11, 14, 15, 37, 82, 121, 125, 128, 133, 135, 139, 140, 153, 188
Pituitary 29, 64, 66, 197, 199, 212
Plasticizers 143, 218
Plastics 121, 125, 126, 134, 143
PMS 62, 63
Pollution 9, 45, 127, 134, 138, 139, 142, 218

Pregnenolone 29, 47, 48, 49, 50, 51, 60, 63, 71, 91
Pregnenolone Steal 47, 48, 49, 50, 51, 60, 71, 91
Prevention 20, 33, 37, 39, 56, 156, 203, 222
Progesterone 29, 47, 49, 50, 63, 67, 192
Protein 16, 66, 79, 86, 87, 88, 97, 175, 176, 177, 179, 180, 181, 183, 188, 213

R

Radiation xv, 19, 38, 45, 69, 149, 150, 151, 152, 154, 156, 157, 158, 159, 160, 161, 207, 219
Reverse osmosis 142, 186

S

Salivary testing 48
Saunas 15, 131, 146, 147
Secretory immunoglobulins 52, 65
Shellfish 121, 128
Sleep xiv, 11, 16, 33, 34, 37, 44, 45, 48, 49, 50, 62, 66, 83, 98, 122, 155, 156, 157, 159, 166, 173, 174, 190, 192, 193, 194, 195, 221, 222
Soy 84, 87, 88, 89, 114, 213
Soy protein isolate 213
Stachybotrys chartarum 112, 114
Stress iii, vii, ix, xiv, xvii, xviii, xix, 1, xiii, xiii, 13, 13, xiii, xiv, xviii, 9, 11, 14, 16, 18, 19, 20, 25, 19, 13, iii, 13, 17, 18, 19, 20, 22, 31, 37, 43, 44, 46, 47, 49, 51, 52, 53, 54, 57, 60, 63, 73, 77, 80, 103, 110, 130, 132, 133, 143, 144, 147, 151, 159, 163, 166, 174, 192, 198, 199, 200, 209, 21, 221, 28, 206, 222, 219, 222, 44, 25, 26, 27, 29, 32, 33, 34, 37, 38, 39, 43, 44, 220, 104, 44, 45, 46, 47, 48, 49, 50, 51, 53, 56, 60, 61, 64, 67, 70, 71, 72, 75, 79, 80, 84, 86, 91, 93, 96, 102, 103, 109, 111, 118, 119, 123, 130, 134, 138, 144, 145, 147, 151, 153, 154, 155, 158, 159, 160, 161, 164, 165, 167, 168, 169, 170, 173, 174, 185, 191, 192, 195, 197, 199, 200, 201, 202, 203, 217, 219, 221
Stress management 16, 33, 34, 37, 167, 174
Stress, situational 43, 173
Stress, subclinical 39, 44
Subclinical 21, 33, 37, 38, 39, 40, 41, 44, 50, 61, 75, 80, 81, 89, 165
Subclinical gluten intolerance 50, 80, 81, 89
Sucrose 45, 84, 97
sucrose intolerance 45, 97
Sulfhydryl groups 145

T

Testosterone 29, 47, 49, 192
Toxic products 134
Toxoplasma gondii 104
Trans-fats 184
Trauma 45, 163, 164, 165, 166, 168, 169, 170, 220

V

Villi 73, 84, 85
Viruses 29, 44, 53, 71, 72, 194

W

Water 4, 6, 8, 31, 32, 37, 50, 74, 79, 94, 99, 107, 108, 111, 112, 114, 116, 117, 118, 125, 126, 127, 128, 130, 134, 135, 139, 140, 141, 142, 143, 144, 145, 157, 160, 182, 183, 186, 188, 190, 191, 196, 198, 214, 216
Water filters 107
Water, filtration 108

Weight gain 50, 62, 188
Wheat 73, 79, 81, 89, 176, 177, 178
Whiplash 45, 164

Y

Yeast 53, 54, 55, 71, 86, 93, 98, 102

Z

Zoonotic disease 108

LaVergne, TN USA
07 February 2010
172257LV00003B/2/P